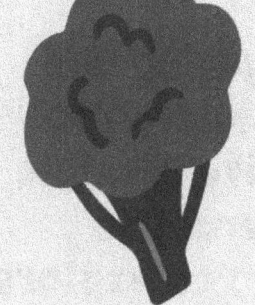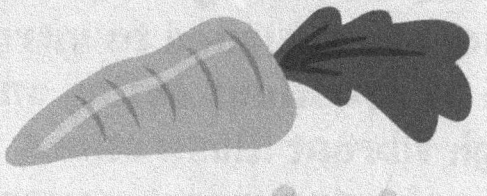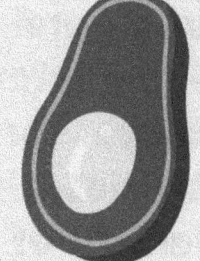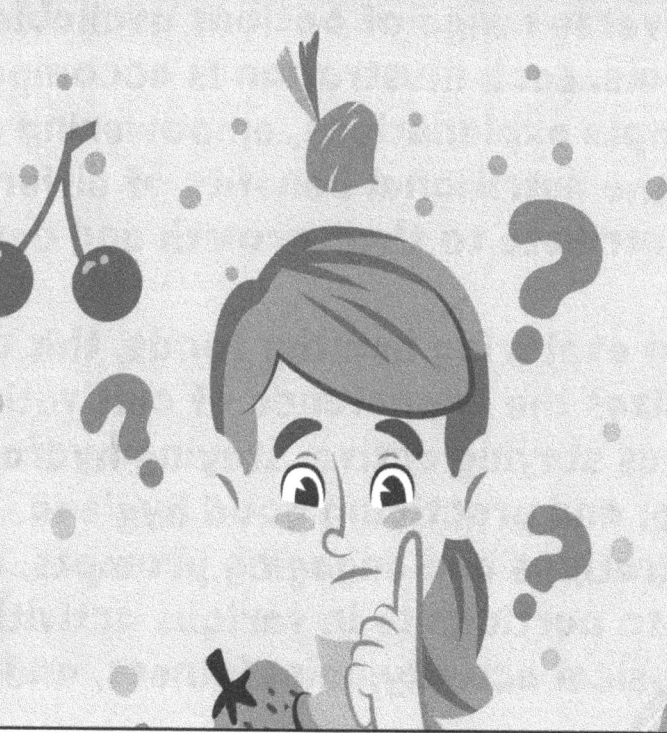

HEALTHY CHOICES COLORING BOOK

THIS BOOK BELONGS TO:
_____

"Healthy Choices Coloring Book" is an engaging and educational resource designed to introduce children to the importance of nutritious eating and positive lifestyle choices. Through vibrant illustrations and interactive activities, this book encourages young readers to explore a variety of healthy foods and habits that promote overall well-being.

Within its pages, children will discover a colorful array of fruits, vegetables, whole grains, and lean proteins, showcasing the diverse range of options available for creating balanced meals. Each illustration is accompanied by fun facts and simple explanations, empowering children to learn about the nutritional benefits of different foods and how they contribute to their growth and development.

In addition to exploring healthy foods, this coloring book also emphasizes the importance of cultivating positive habits, such as staying active, staying hydrated, getting enough sleep, and practicing good hygiene. Through playful illustrations and engaging prompts, children are encouraged to participate in various activities that promote physical activity, mindfulness, and self-care.

By fostering an early appreciation for healthy foods and habits, this coloring book aims to instill lifelong habits that will support children in leading happy, healthy lives. Whether used at home or in educational settings, the "Healthy Choices Coloring Book" serves as a valuable tool for promoting health literacy and empowering children to make informed choices about their nutrition and well-being.

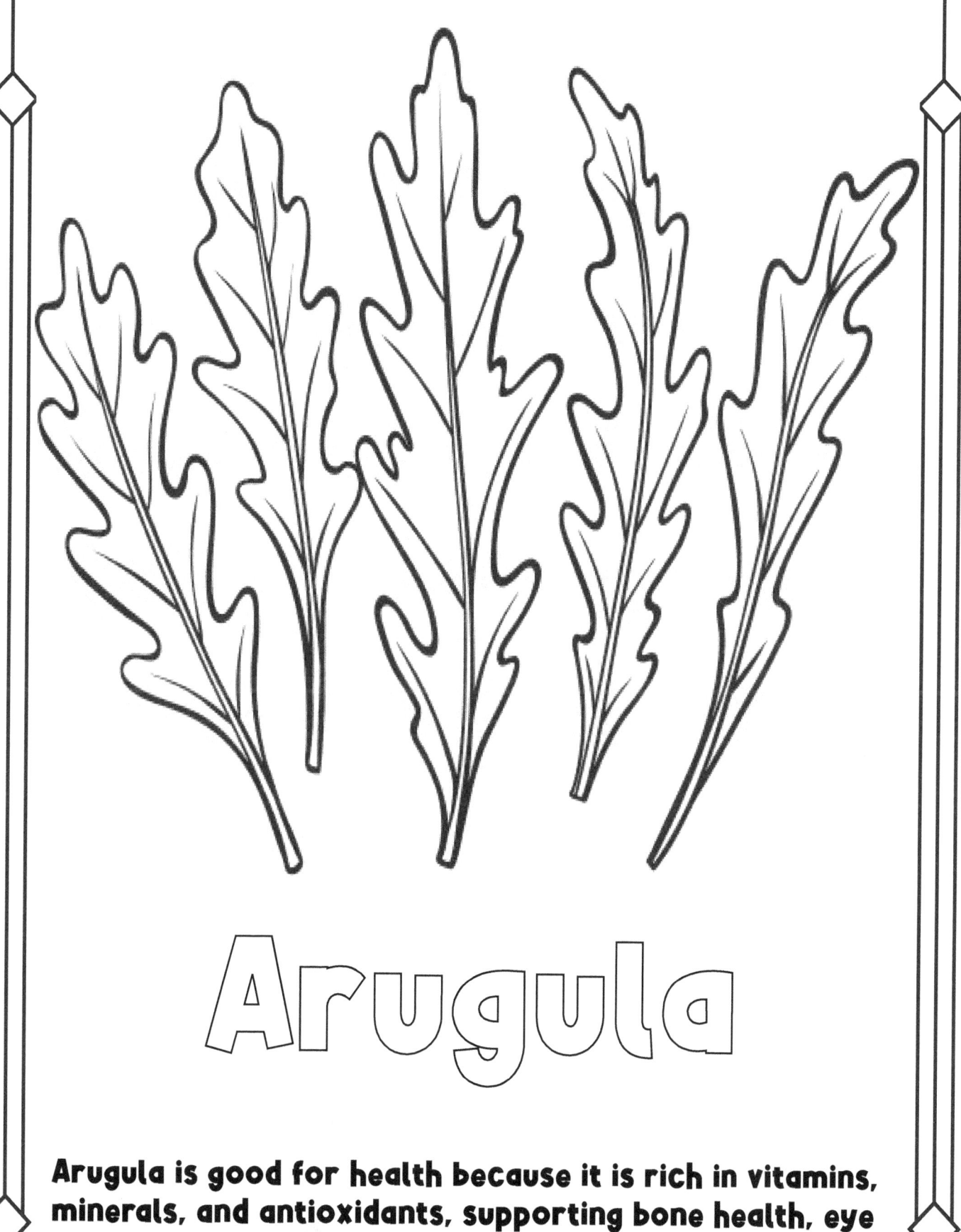

Arugula is good for health because it is rich in vitamins, minerals, and antioxidants, supporting bone health, eye health, and overall immunity.

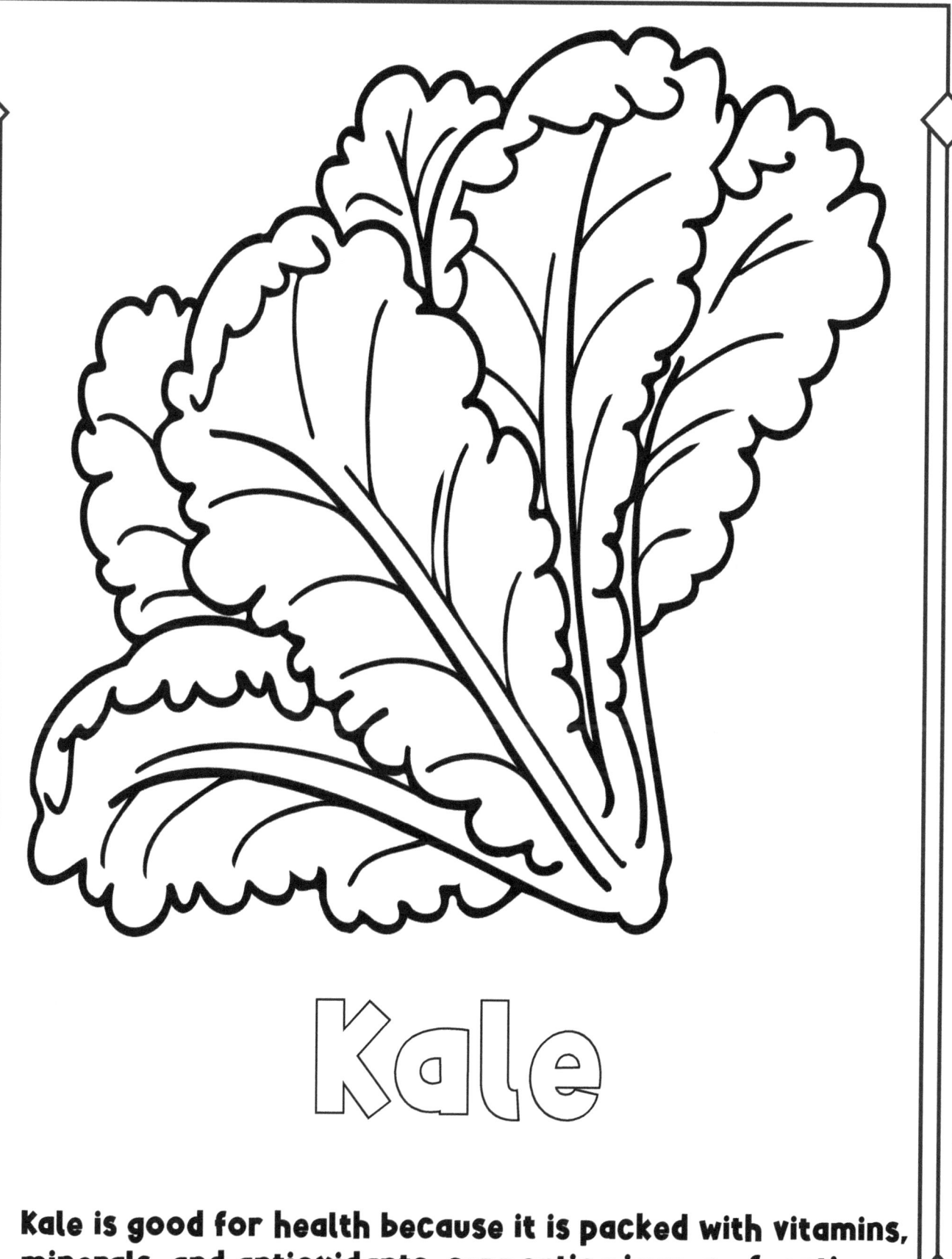

Kale

Kale is good for health because it is packed with vitamins, minerals, and antioxidants, supporting immune function, heart health, and digestion.

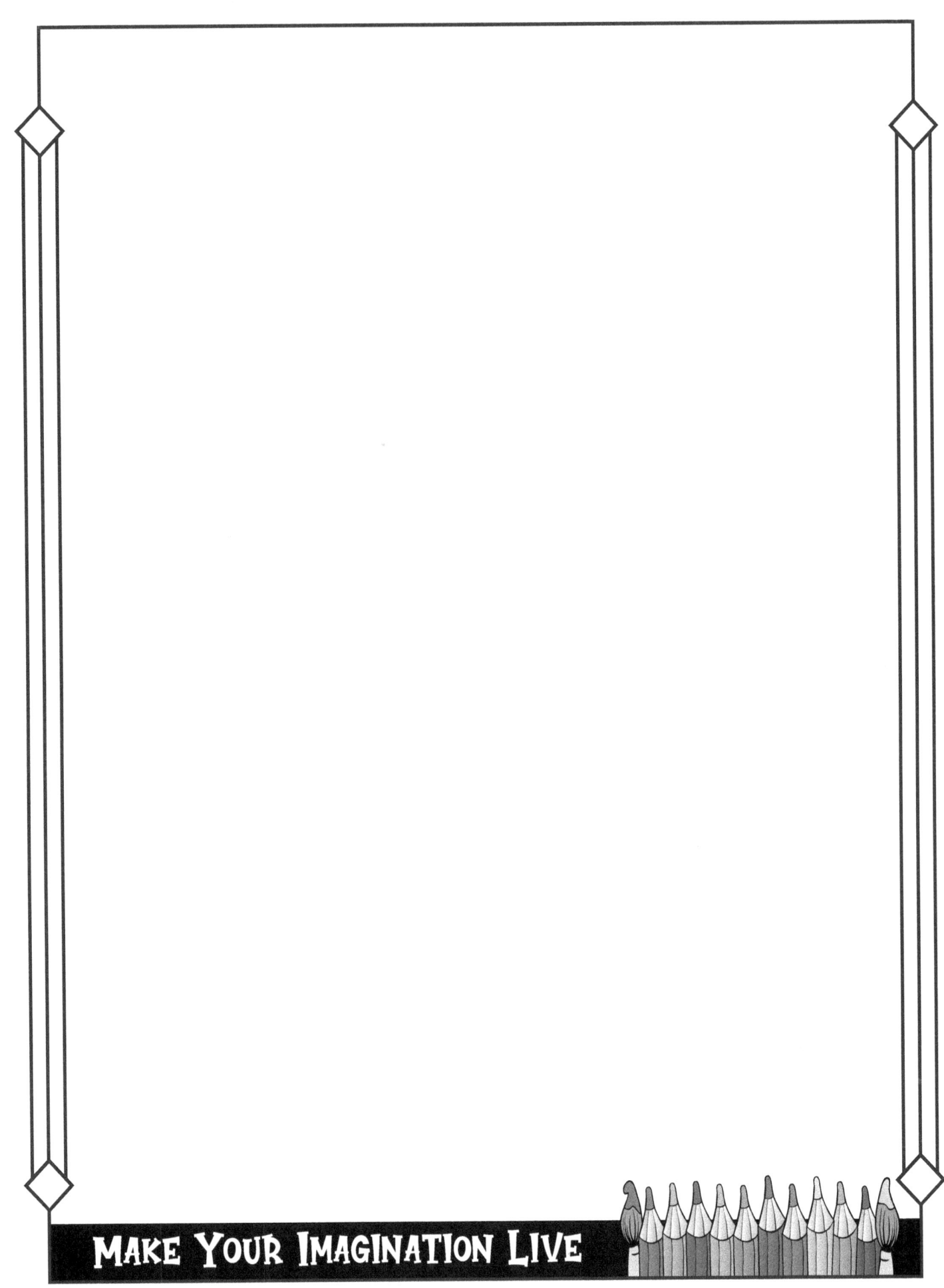

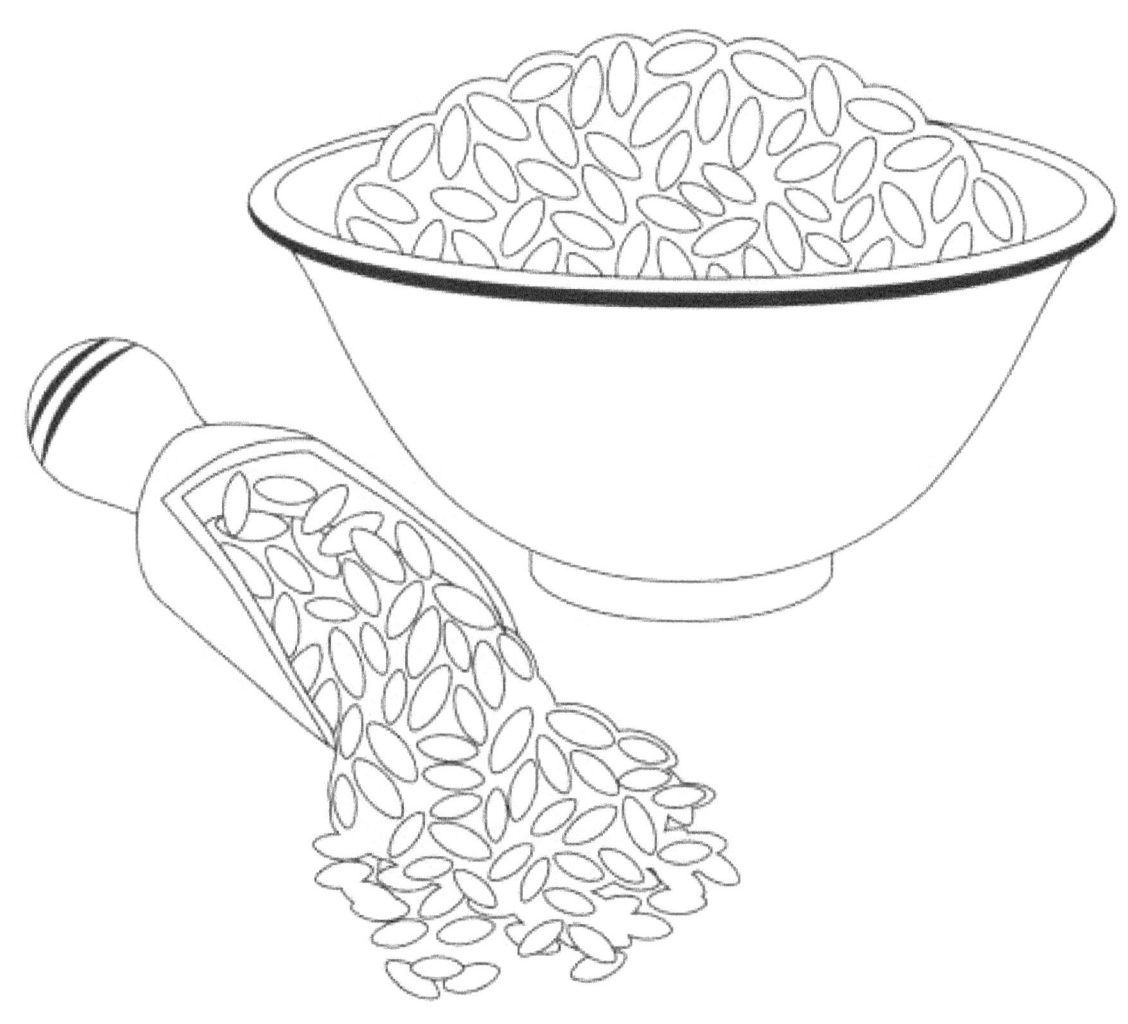

Brown Rice

Brown rice is good for health because it is a whole grain rich in fiber, vitamins, and minerals, supporting digestive health, heart health, and providing sustained energy.

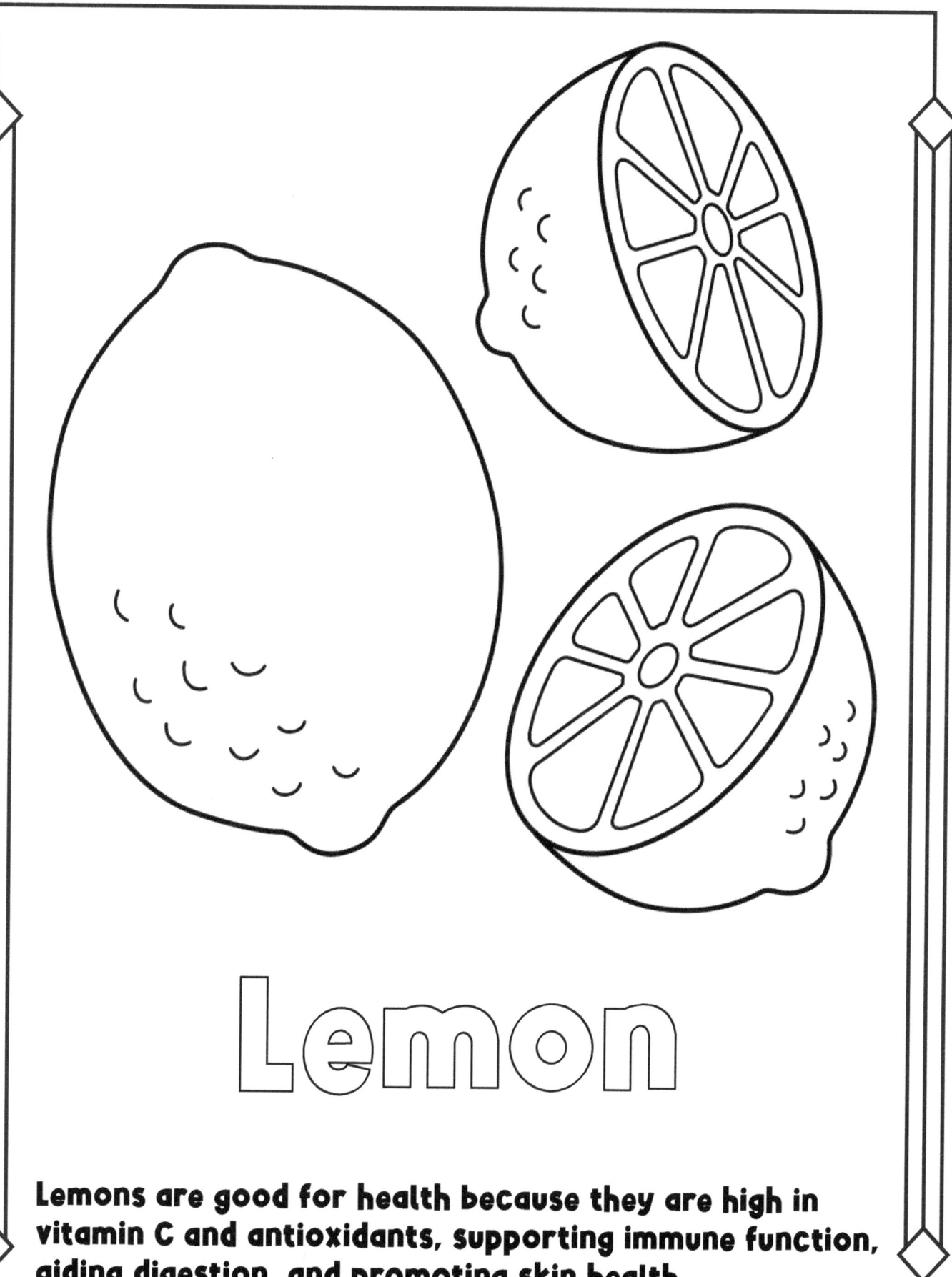

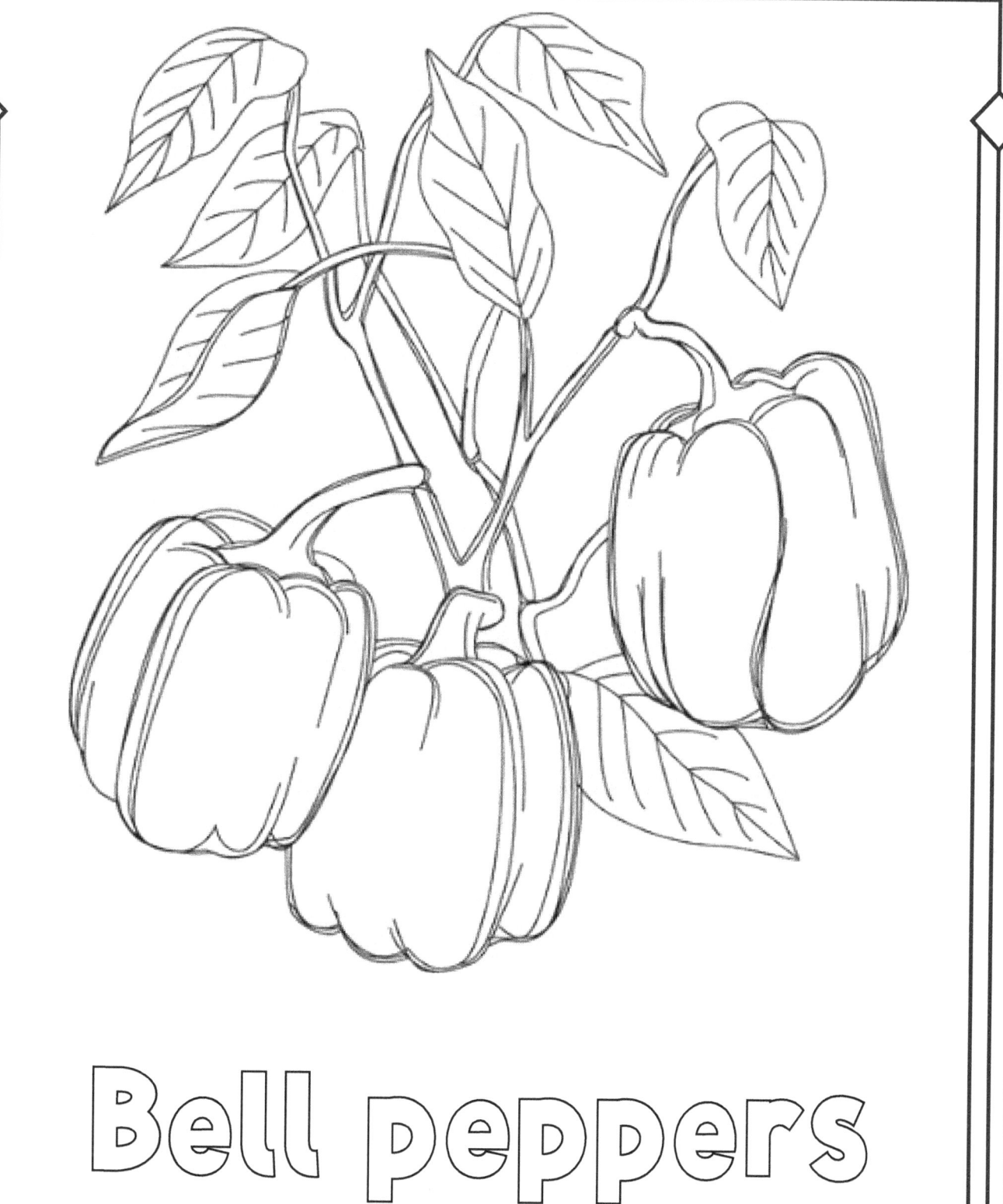

Bell peppers

Bell peppers are good for health because they are rich in vitamins, antioxidants, and fiber, supporting eye health, boosting immunity, and reducing the risk of chronic diseases.

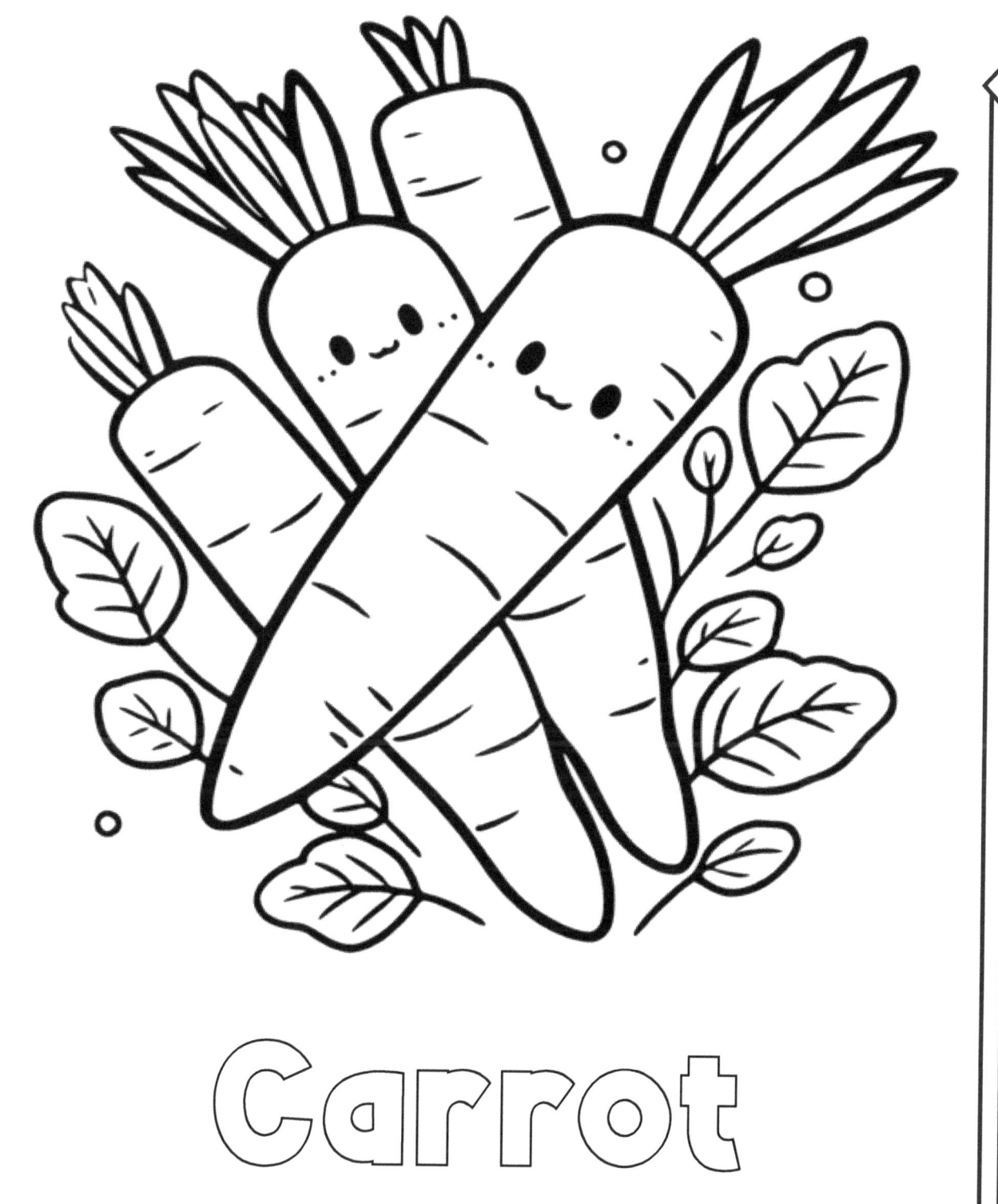

Carrot

Carrots are good for health because they are rich in beta-carotene, fiber, and vitamins, promoting eye health, boosting immunity, and supporting healthy skin.

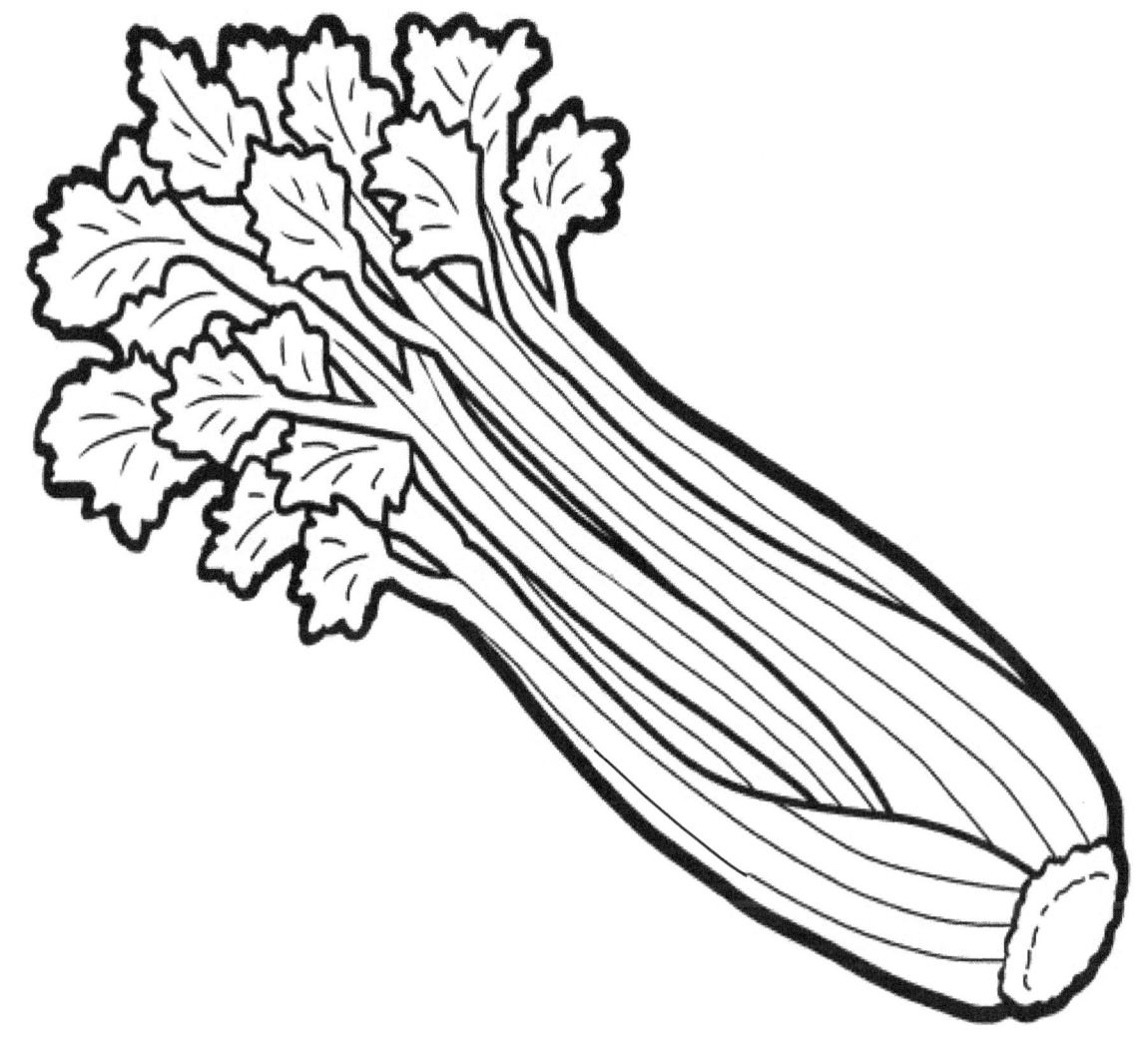

Celery

Celery is good for health because it is low in calories, rich in fiber and antioxidants, supporting digestion, hydration, and heart health.

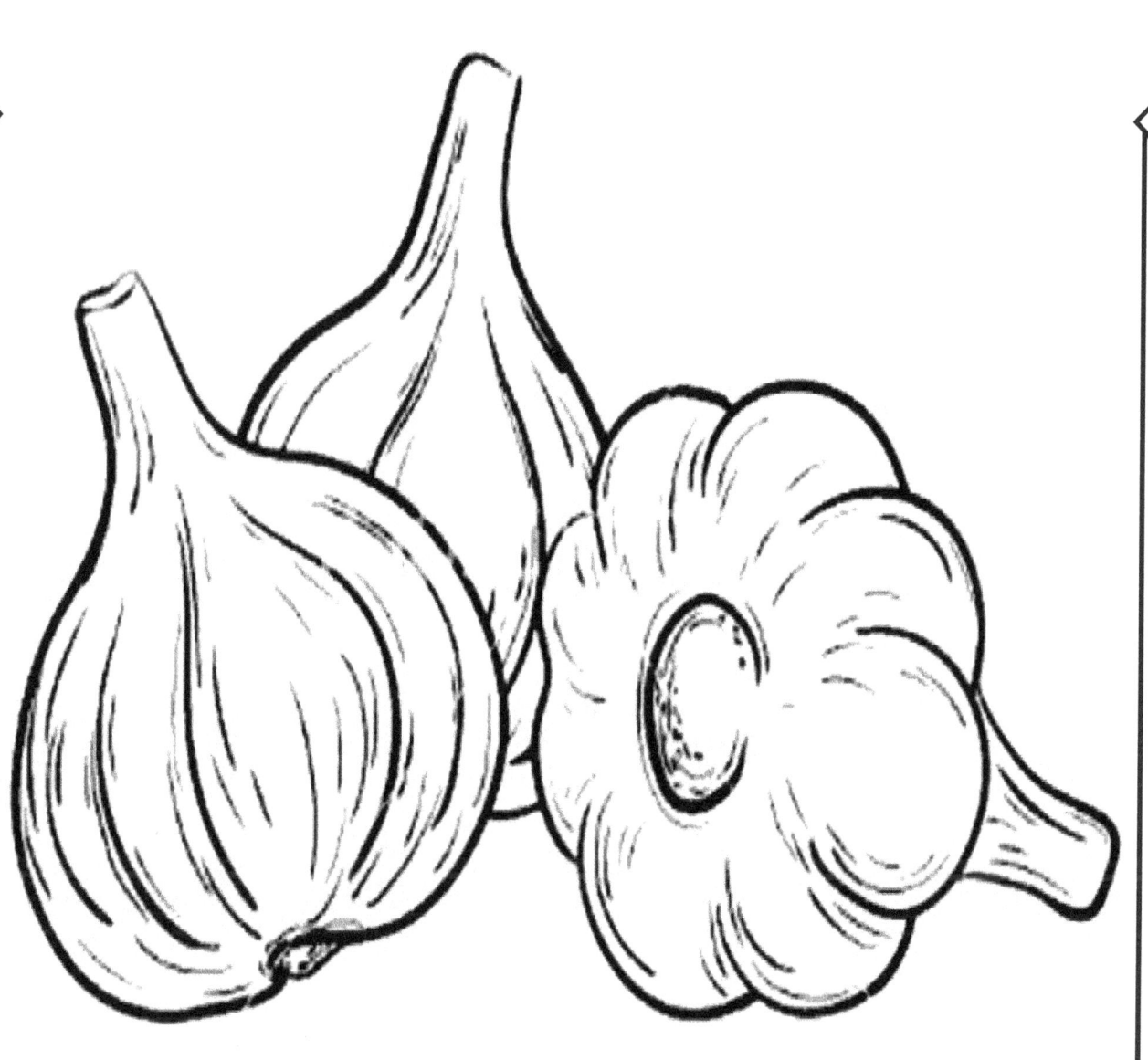

Garlic

Garlic is good for health because it contains compounds that may have various health benefits, including boosting immunity, reducing blood pressure, and supporting heart health.

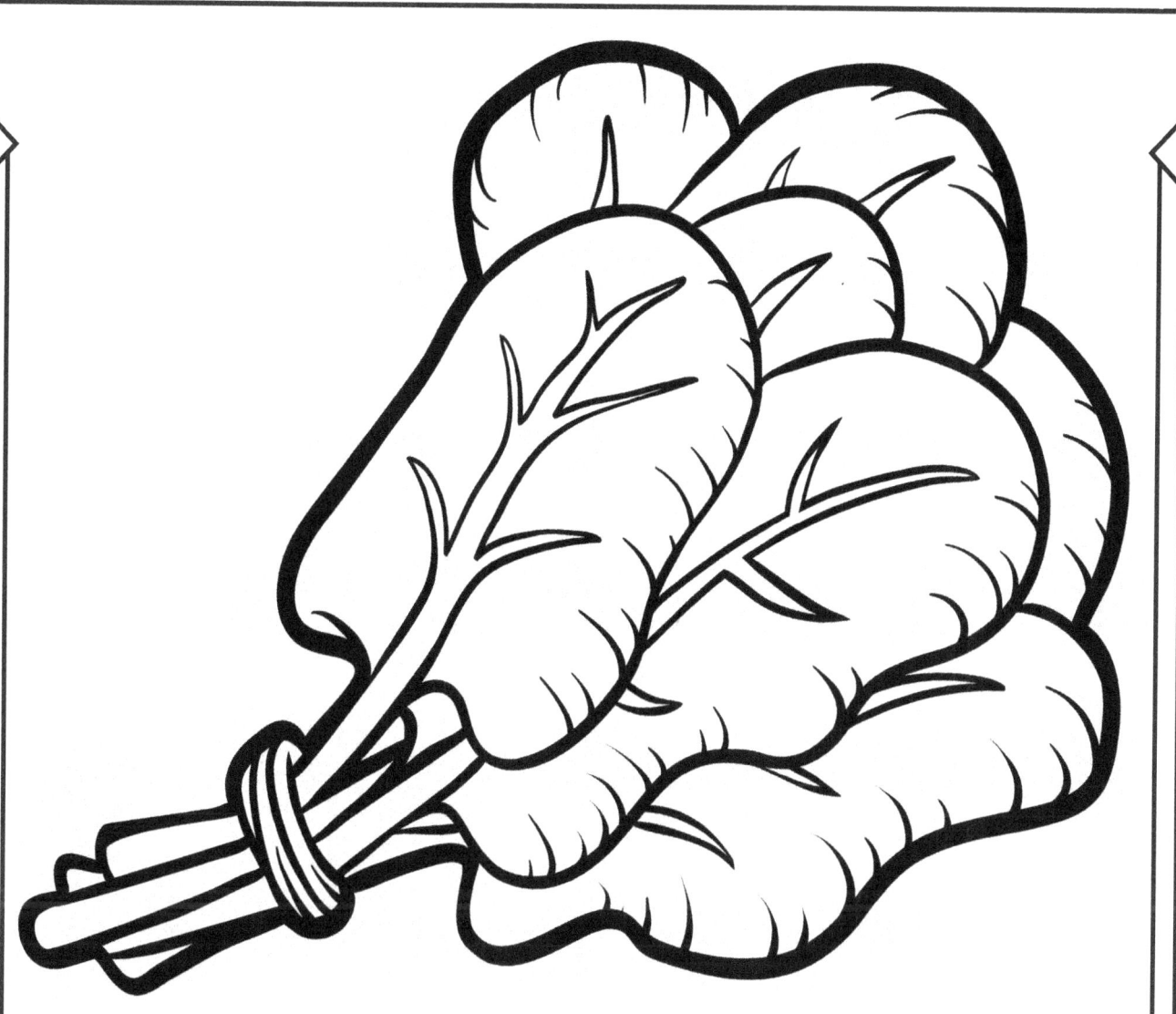

Spinach

Spinach is good for health because it is packed with nutrients like vitamins, minerals, and antioxidants, supporting overall health, including heart health, bone health, and immune function.

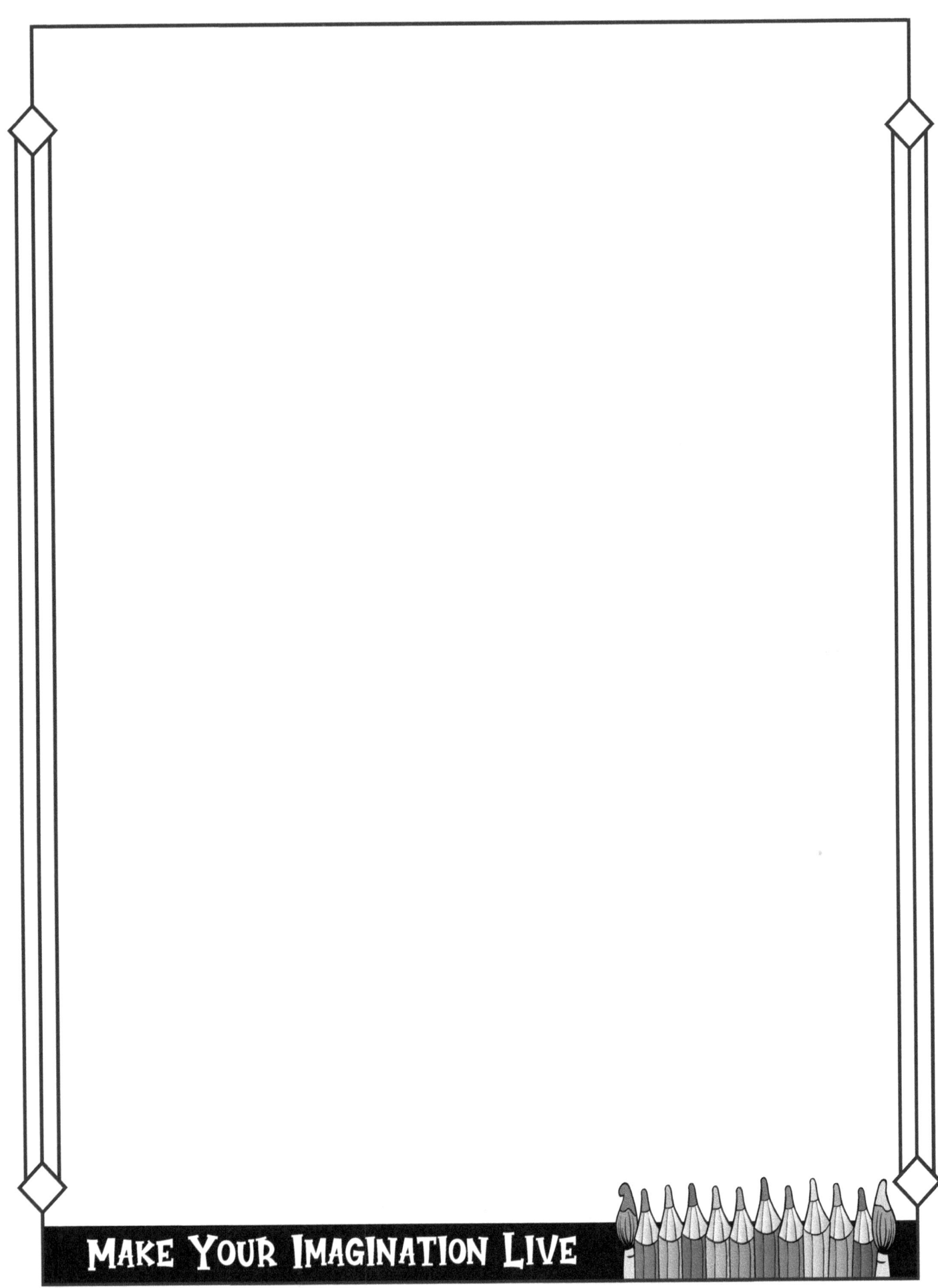

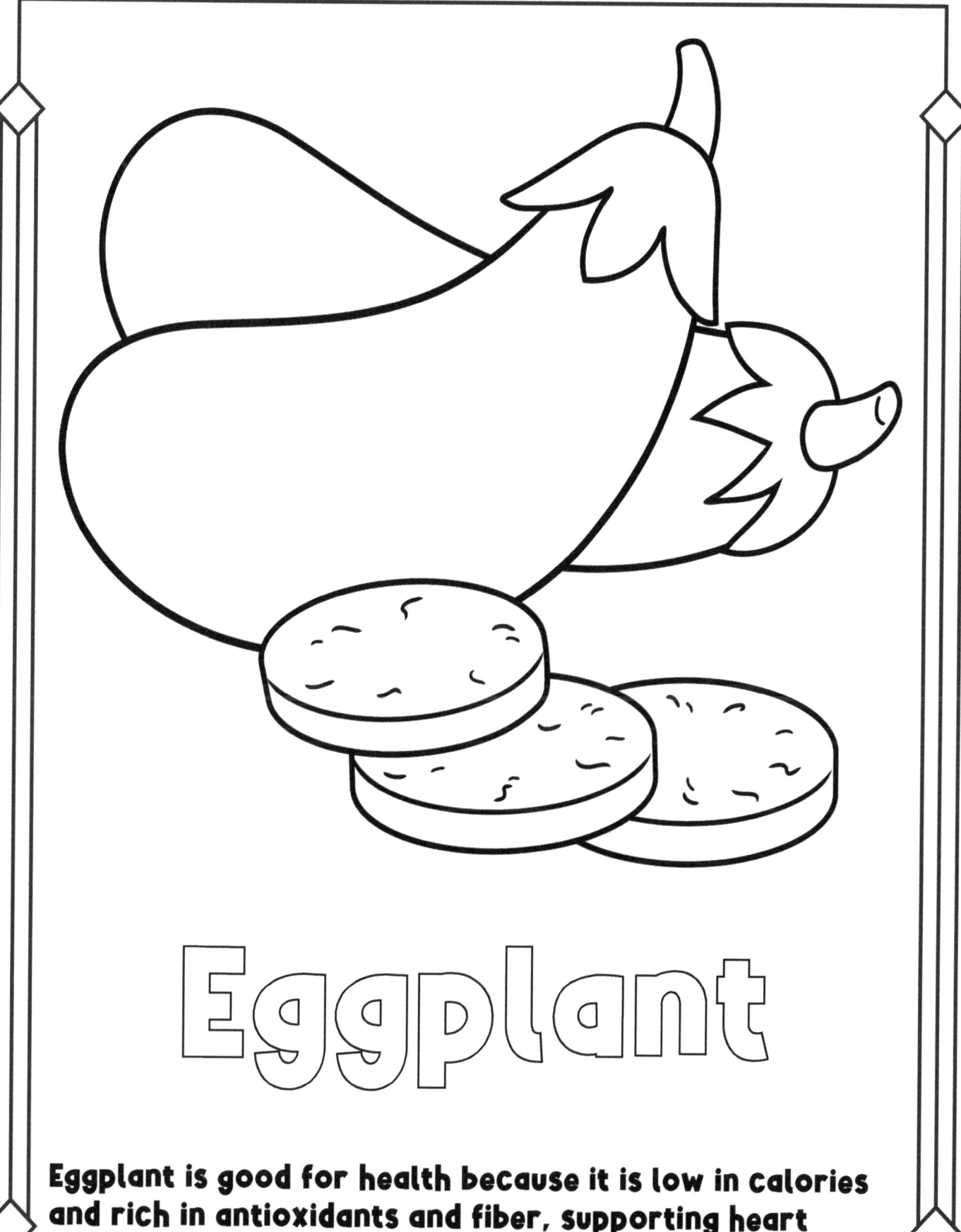

Eggplant

Eggplant is good for health because it is low in calories and rich in antioxidants and fiber, supporting heart health, aiding digestion, and promoting weight management.

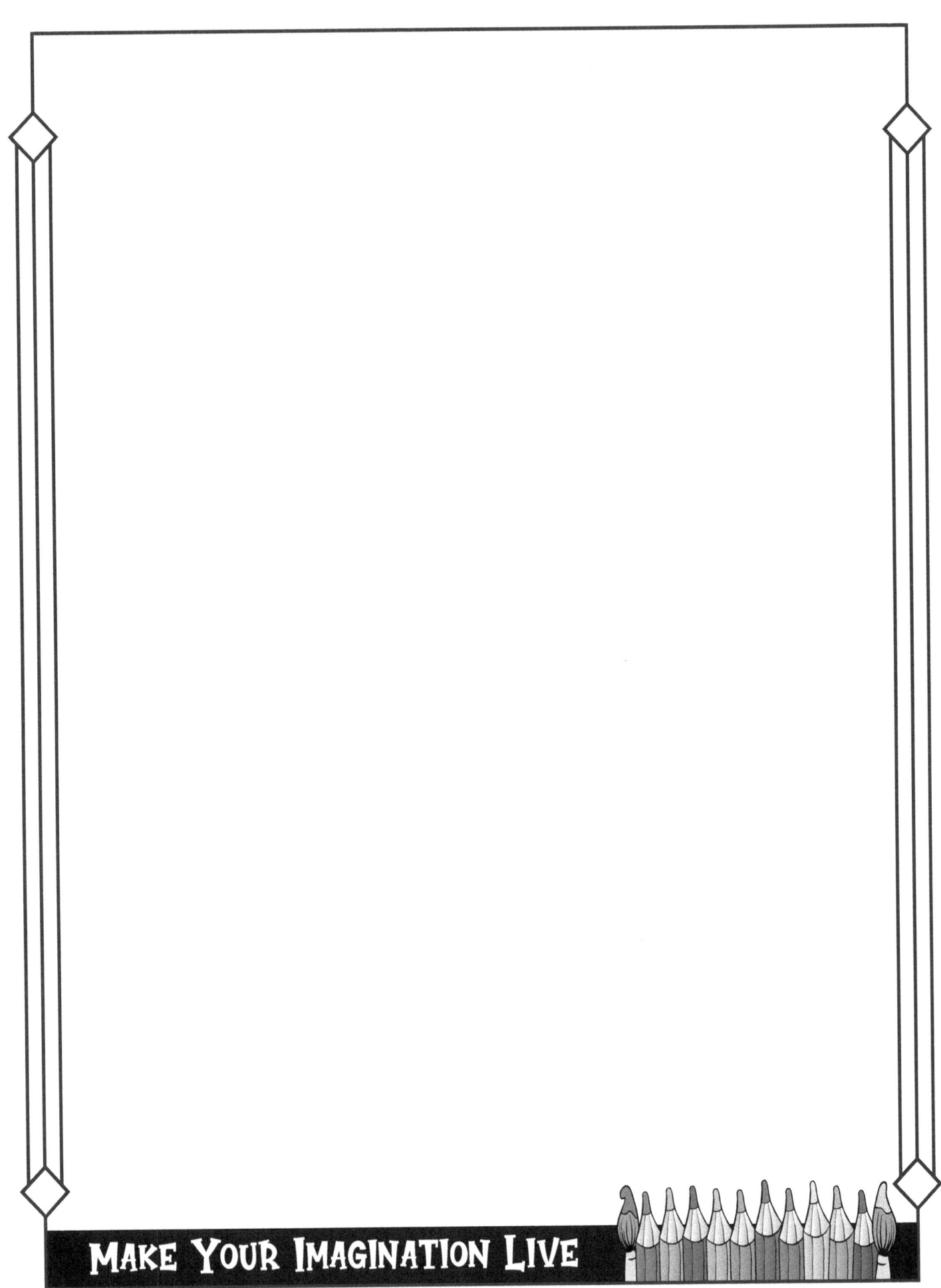

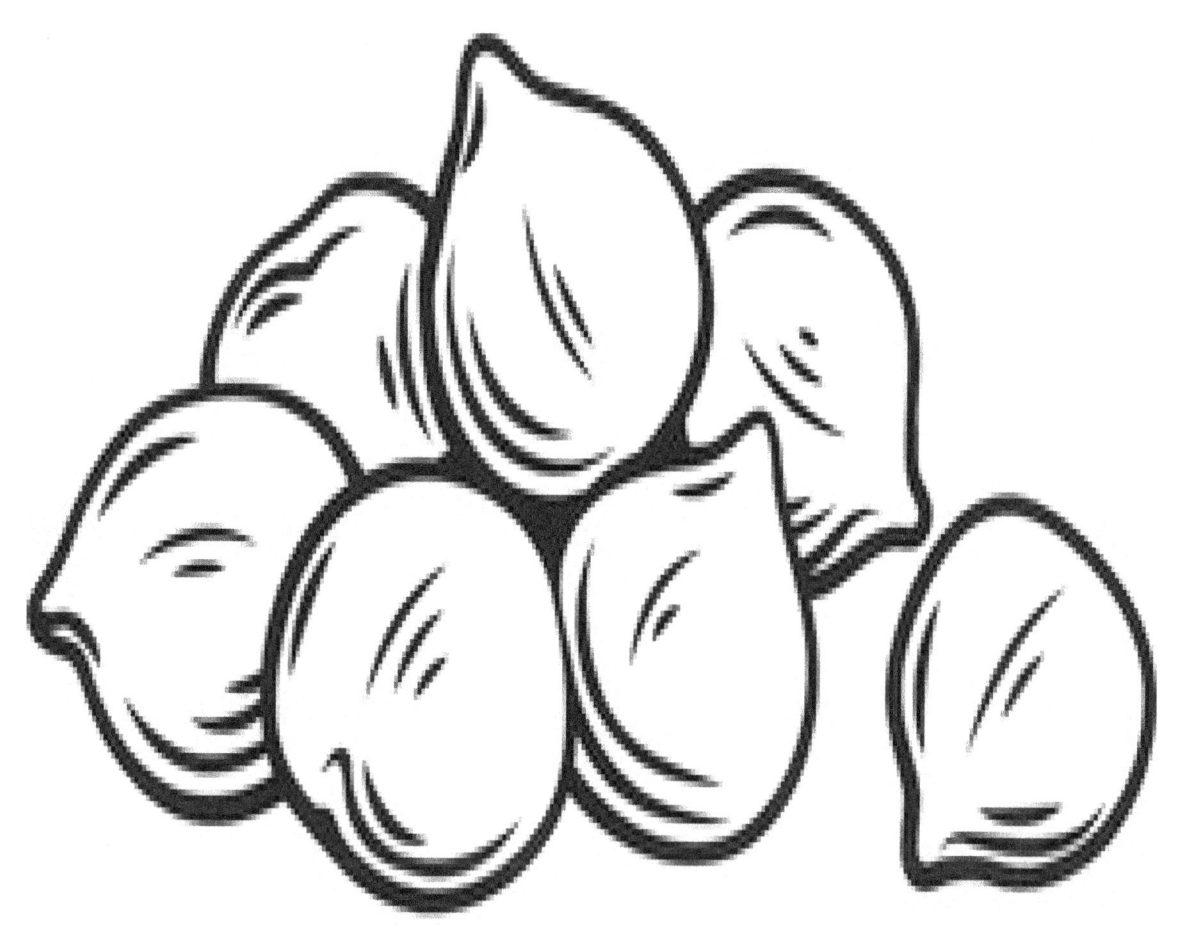

Chickpeas

Chickpeas are good for health because they are high in protein, fiber, and nutrients, supporting digestive health, weight management, and heart health.

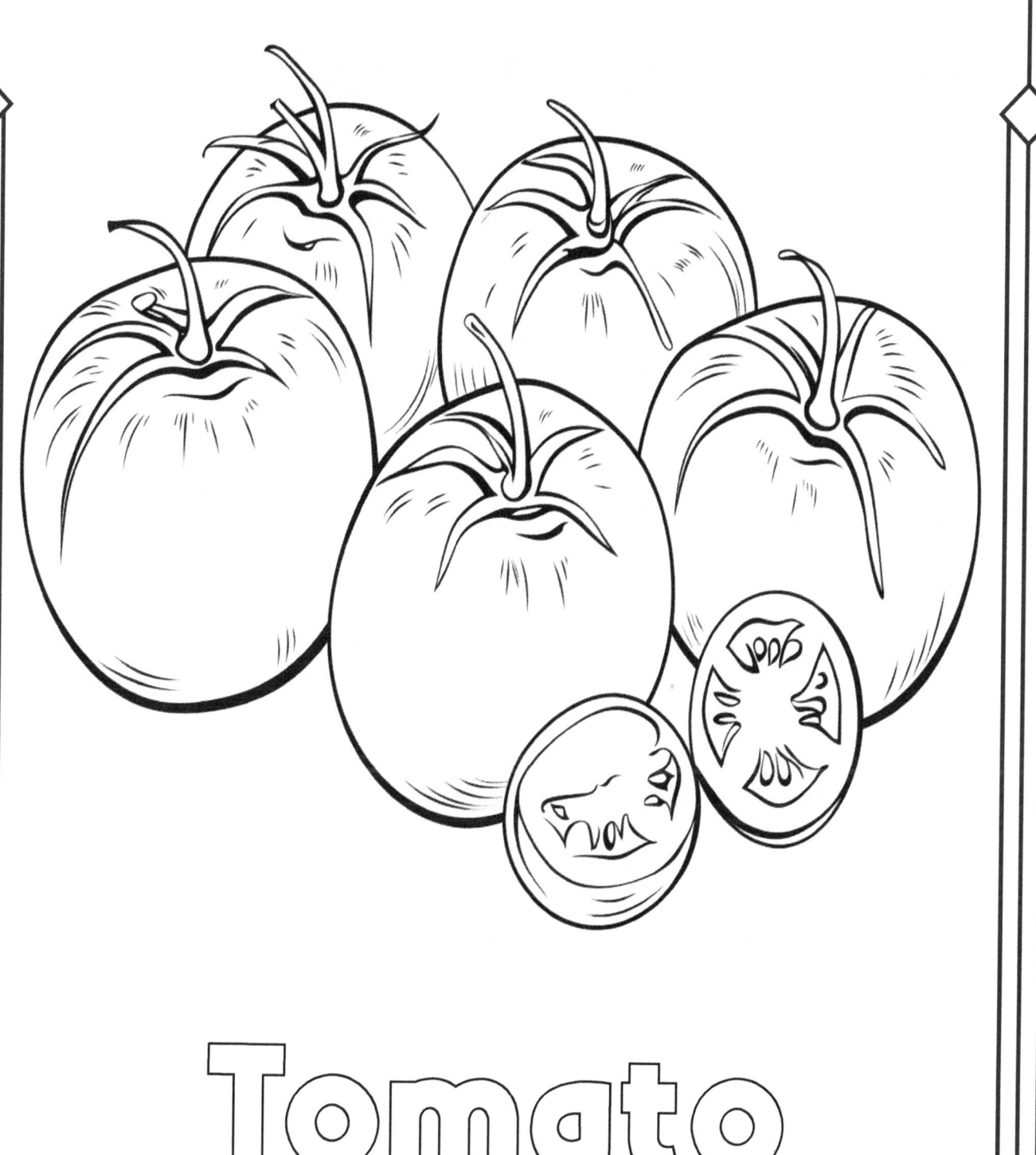

Tomato

Tomatoes are good for health because they are rich in vitamins, minerals, and antioxidants, supporting heart health, eye health, and skin health.

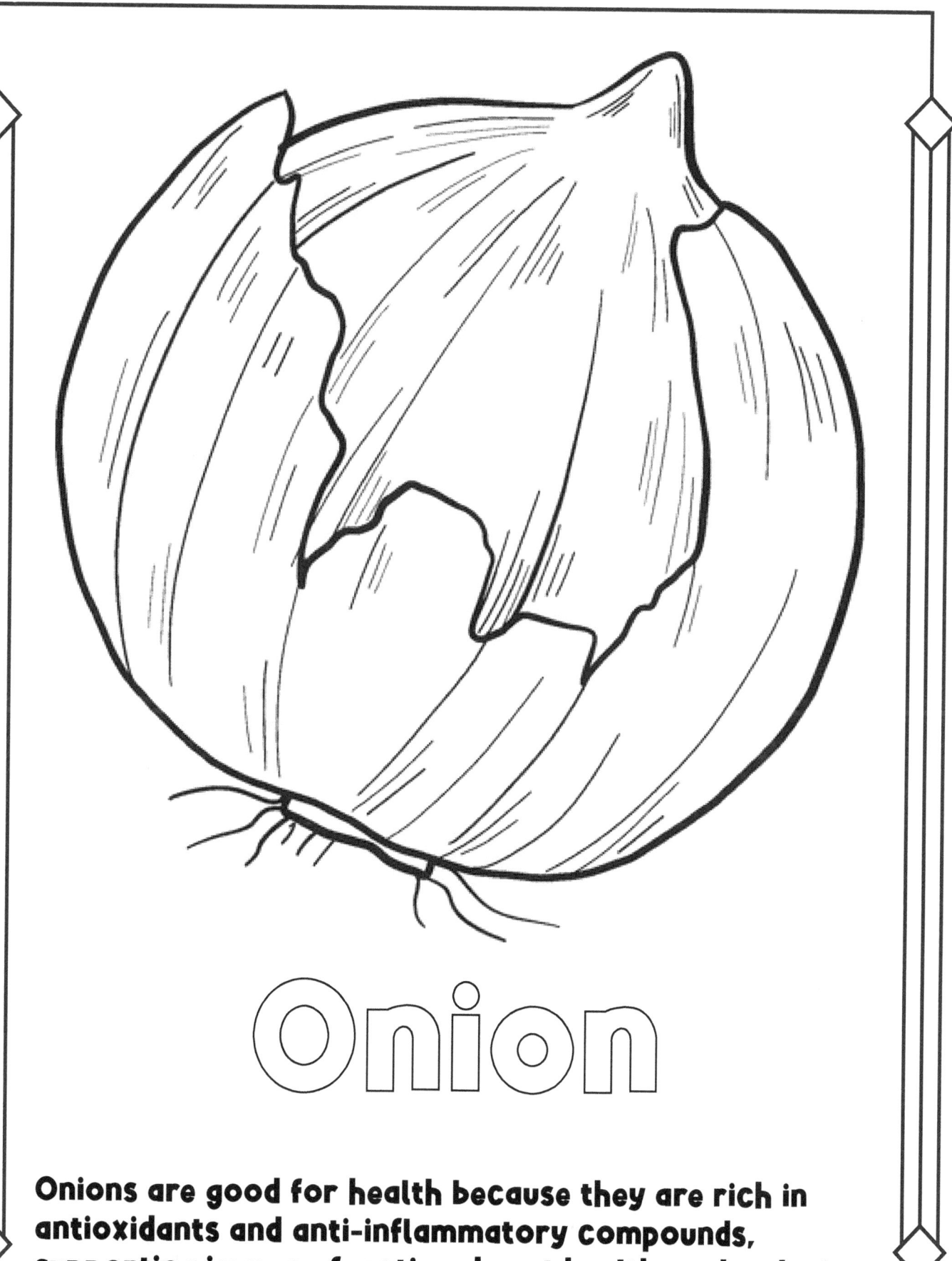

Onion

Onions are good for health because they are rich in antioxidants and anti-inflammatory compounds, supporting immune function, heart health, and reducing the risk of chronic diseases.

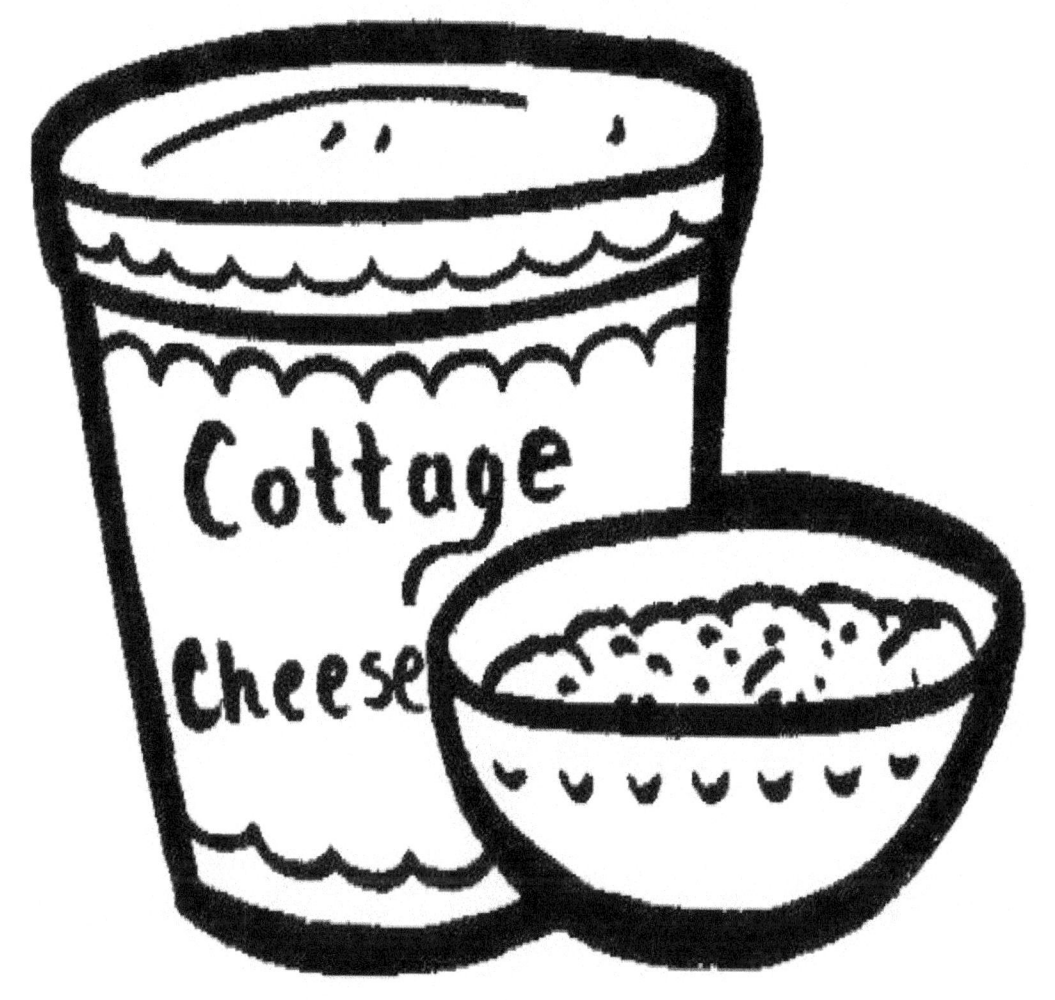

Cottage Cheese

Cottage cheese is good for health because it is high in protein, calcium, and B vitamins, supporting muscle growth, bone health, and weight management.

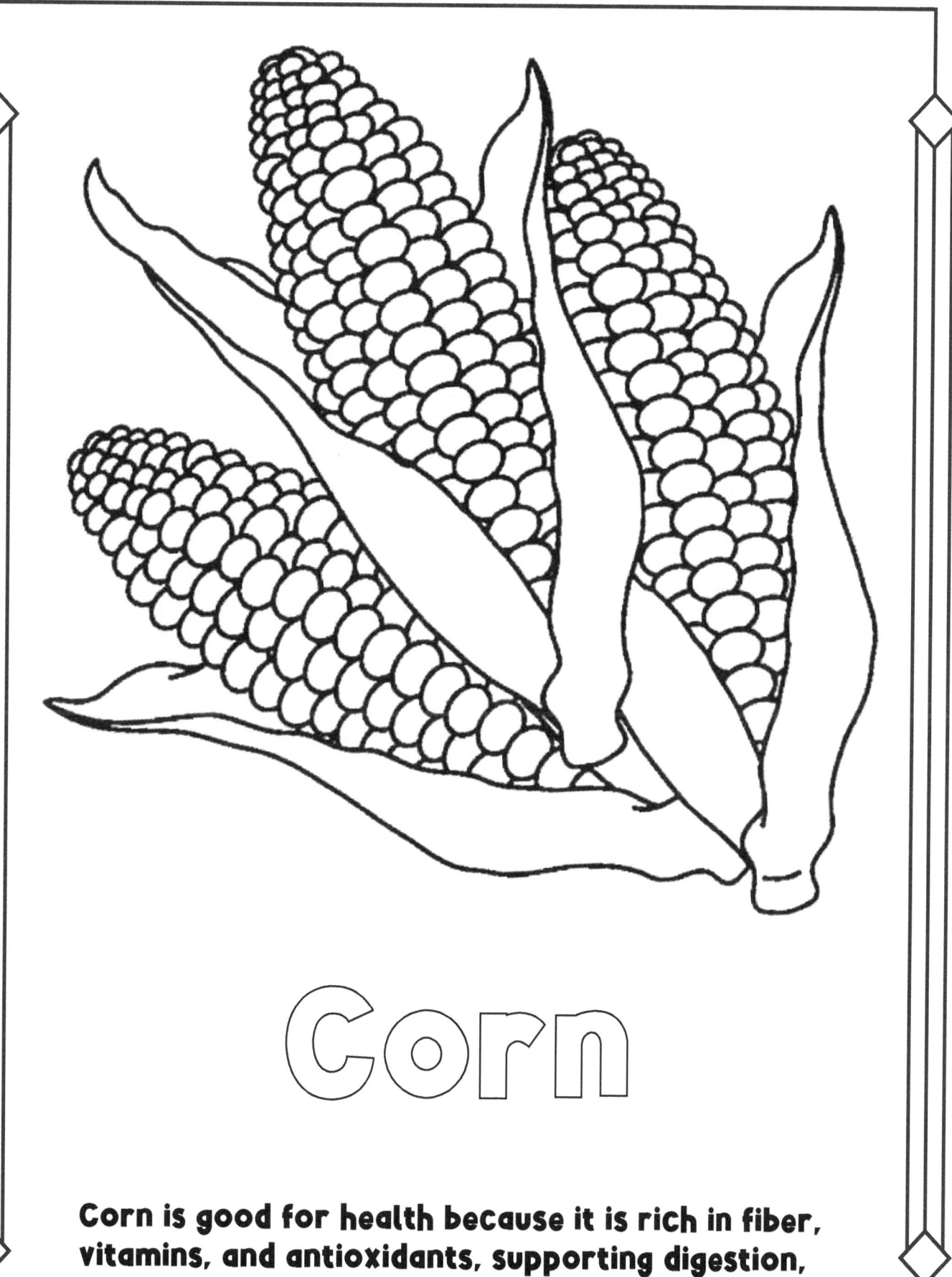

Corn

Corn is good for health because it is rich in fiber, vitamins, and antioxidants, supporting digestion, promoting heart health, and providing energy.

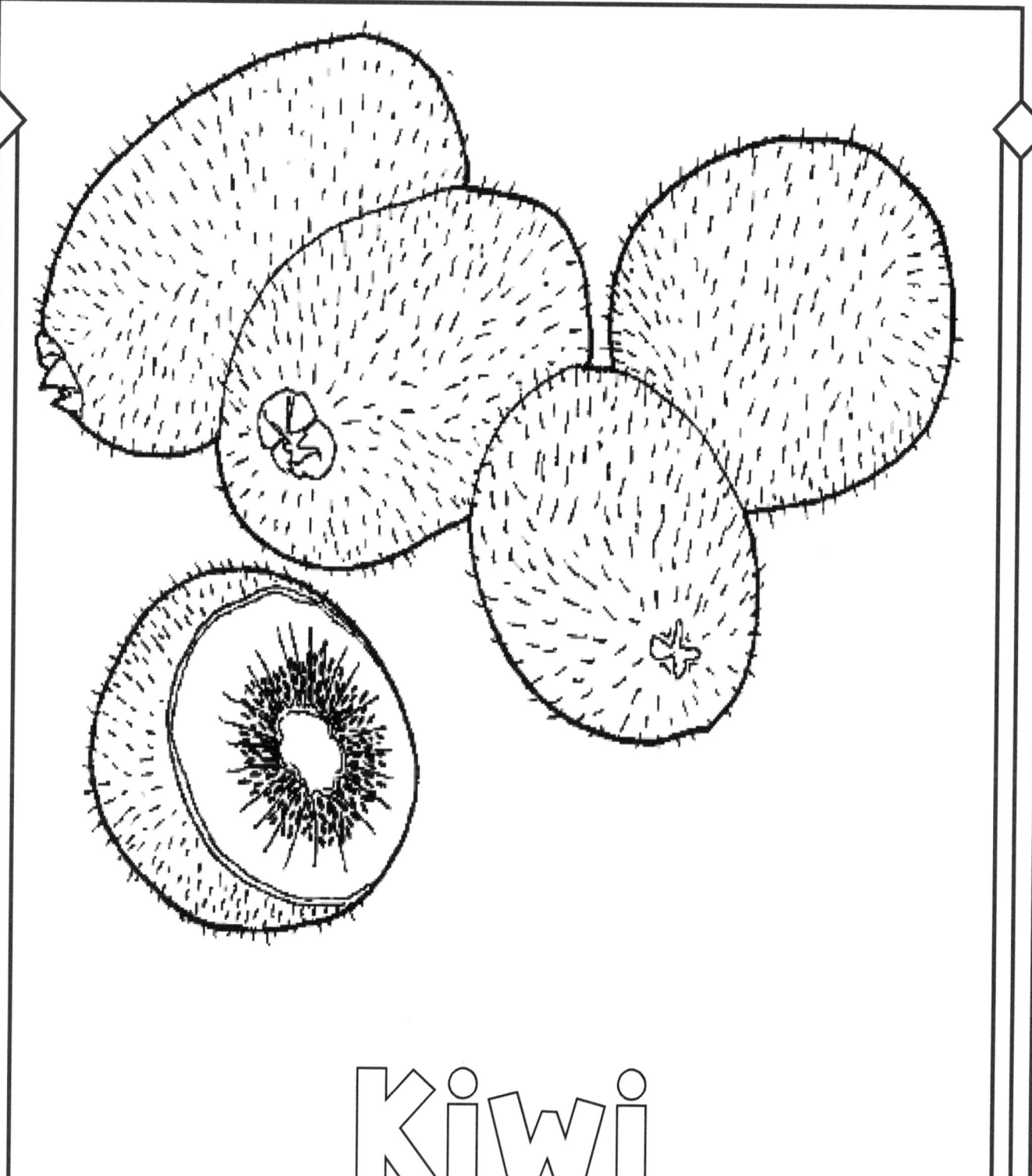

Kiwi

Kiwi is good for health because it is packed with vitamins, minerals, and antioxidants, supporting immune function, aiding digestion, and promoting heart health

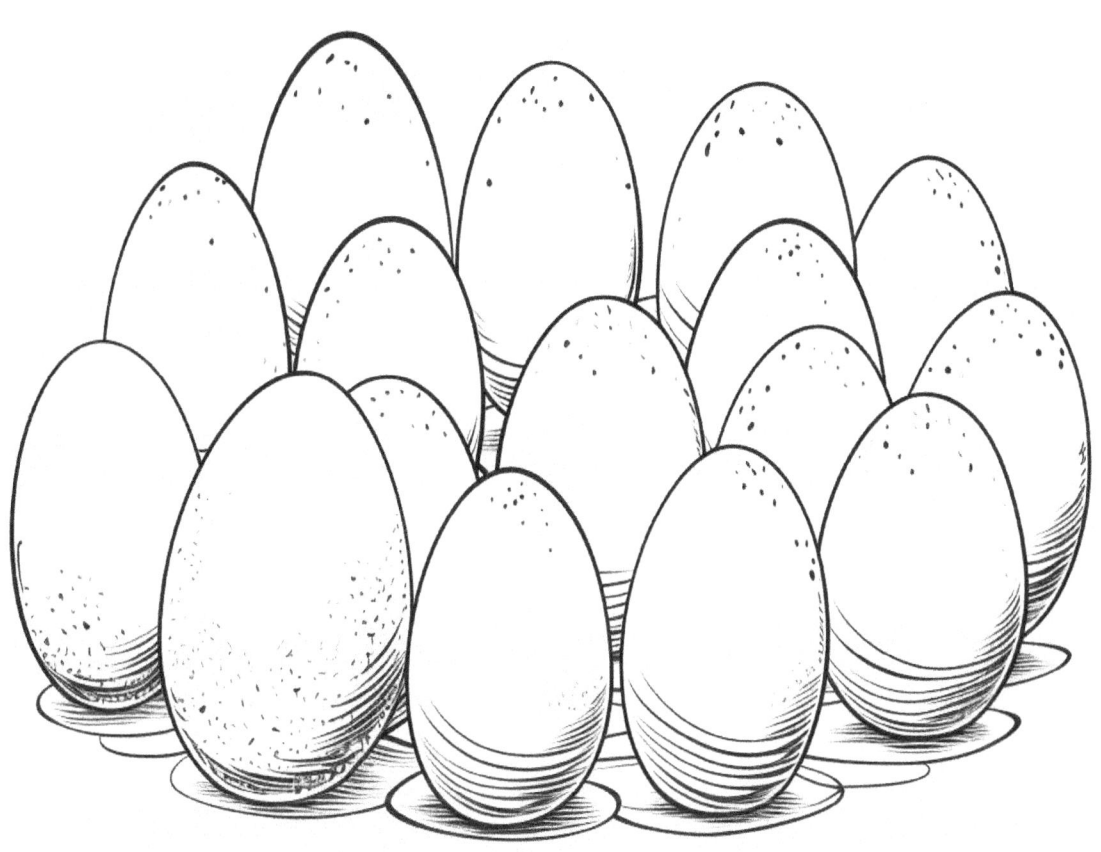

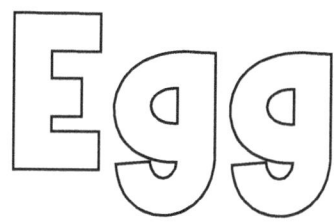

Eggs are good for health because they are a rich source of protein, vitamins, and minerals, supporting muscle development, brain function, and overall health.

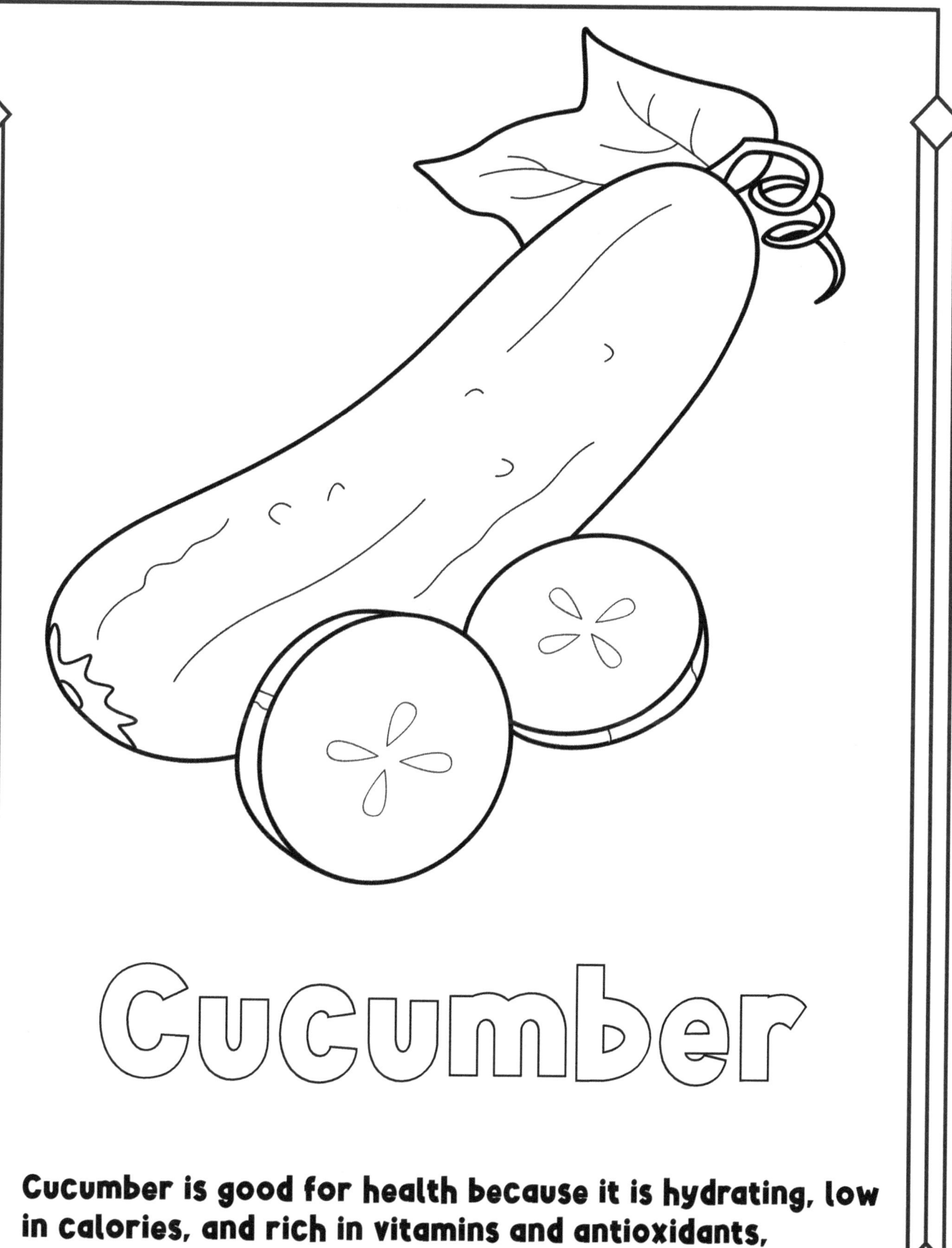

Cucumber

Cucumber is good for health because it is hydrating, low in calories, and rich in vitamins and antioxidants, supporting hydration, aiding digestion, and promoting skin health.

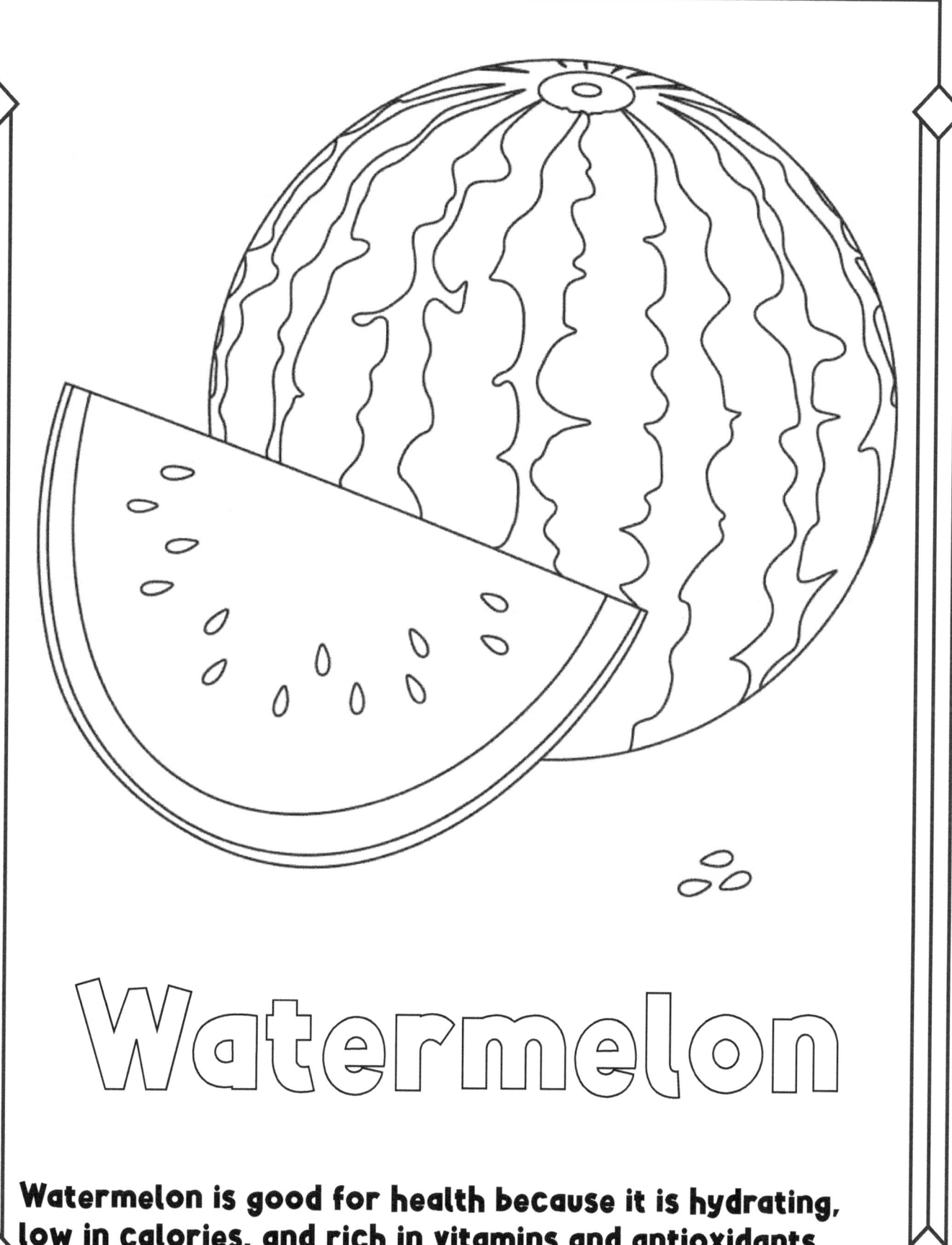

Watermelon

Watermelon is good for health because it is hydrating, low in calories, and rich in vitamins and antioxidants, supporting hydration, promoting heart health, and aiding digestion.

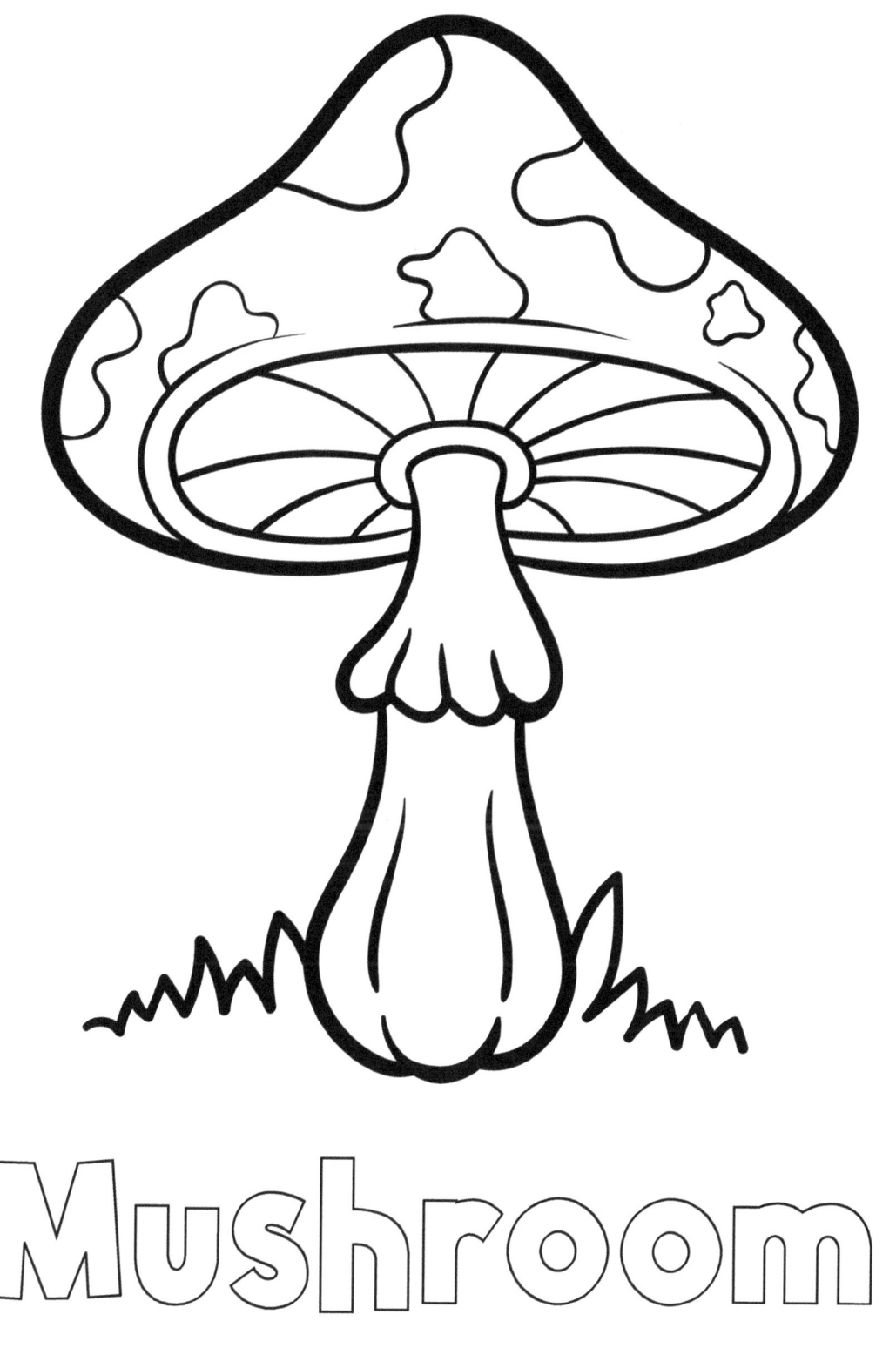

Mushroom

Mushrooms are good for health because they are low in calories and rich in vitamins, minerals, and antioxidants, supporting immune function, heart health, and promoting healthy aging.

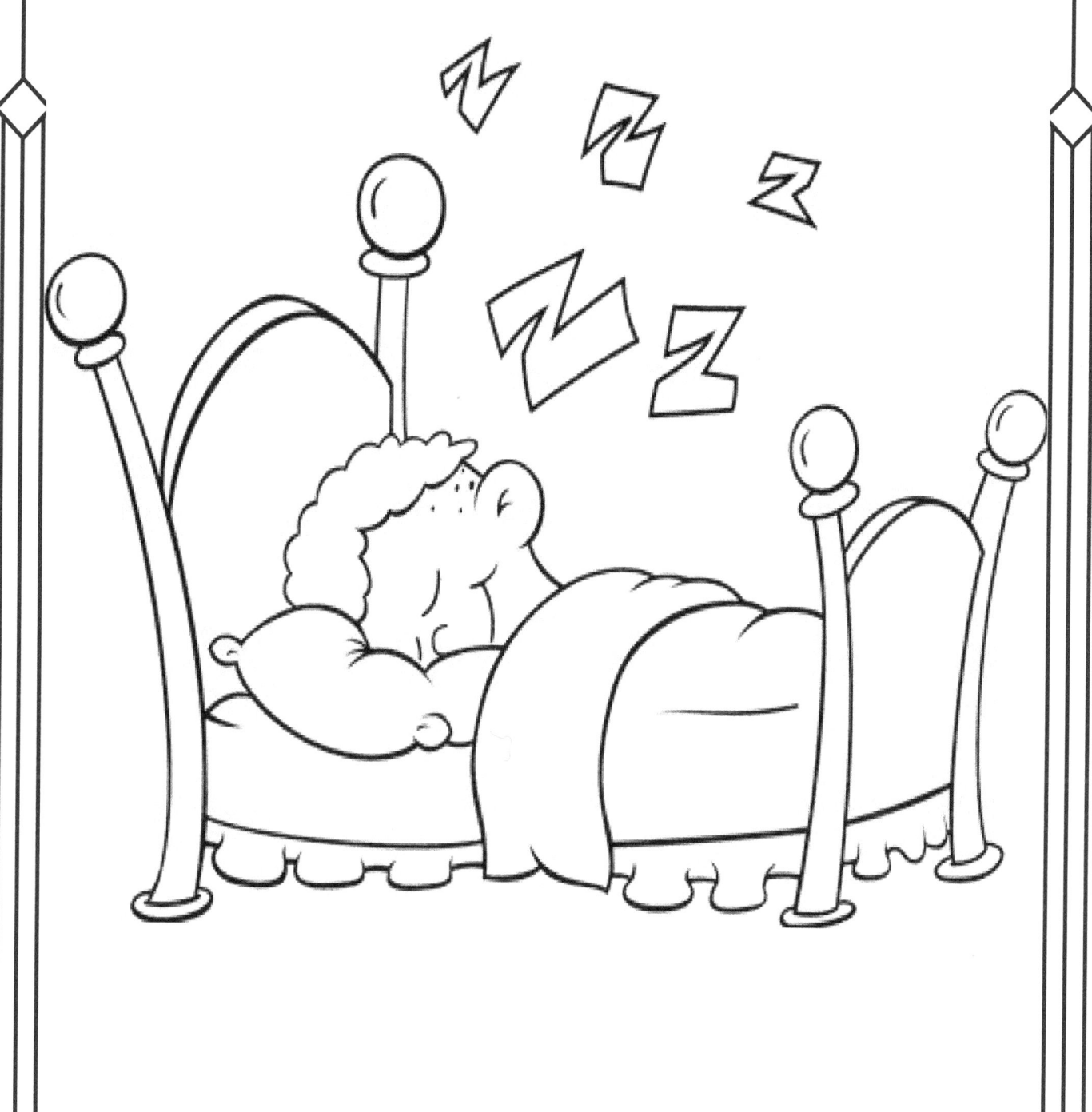

Getting Enough Sleep

Getting enough sleep is good for health because it supports cognitive function, mood regulation, immune function, and overall physical and mental well-being.

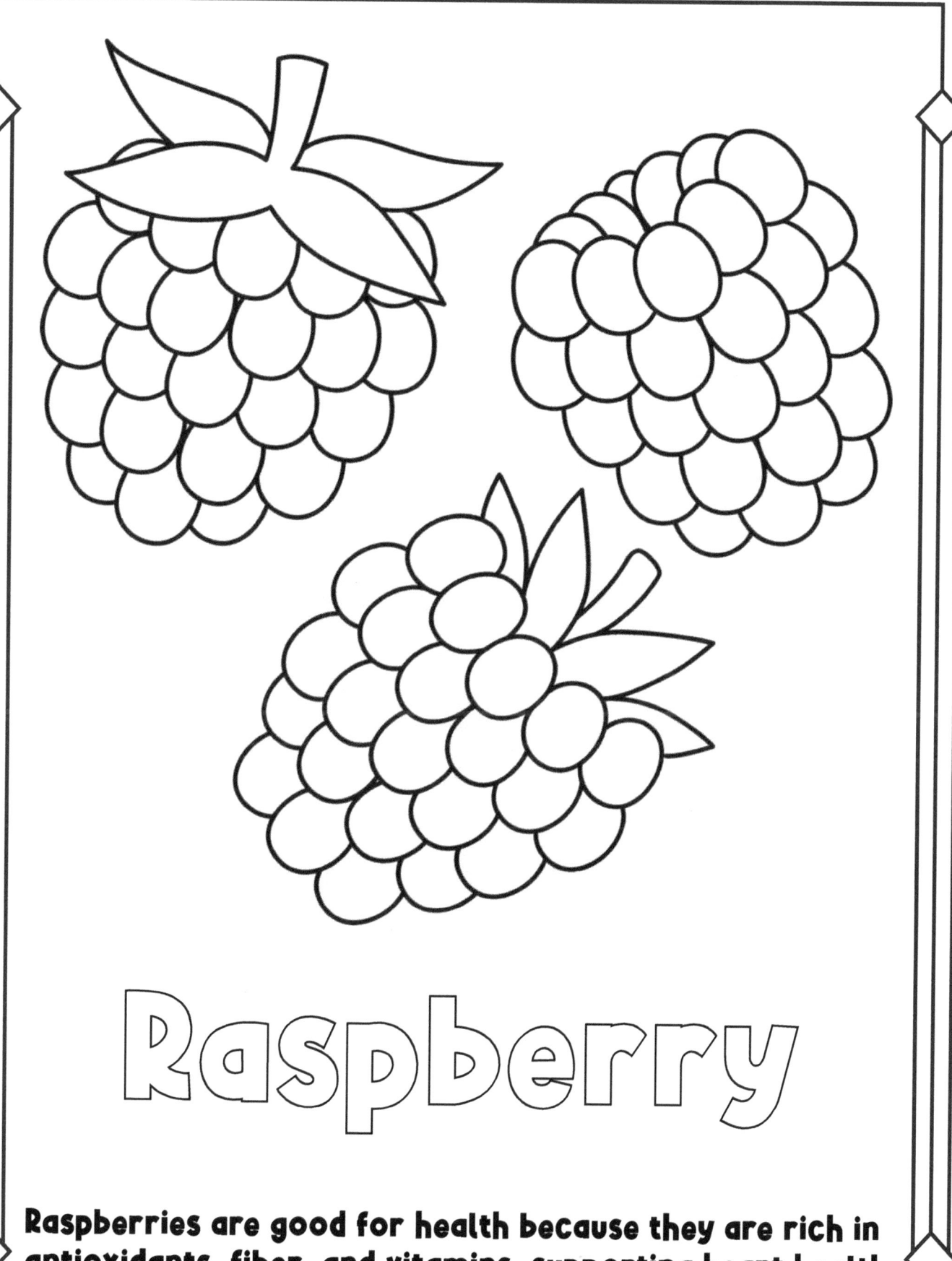

Raspberry

Raspberries are good for health because they are rich in antioxidants, fiber, and vitamins, supporting heart health, aiding digestion, and promoting healthy aging.

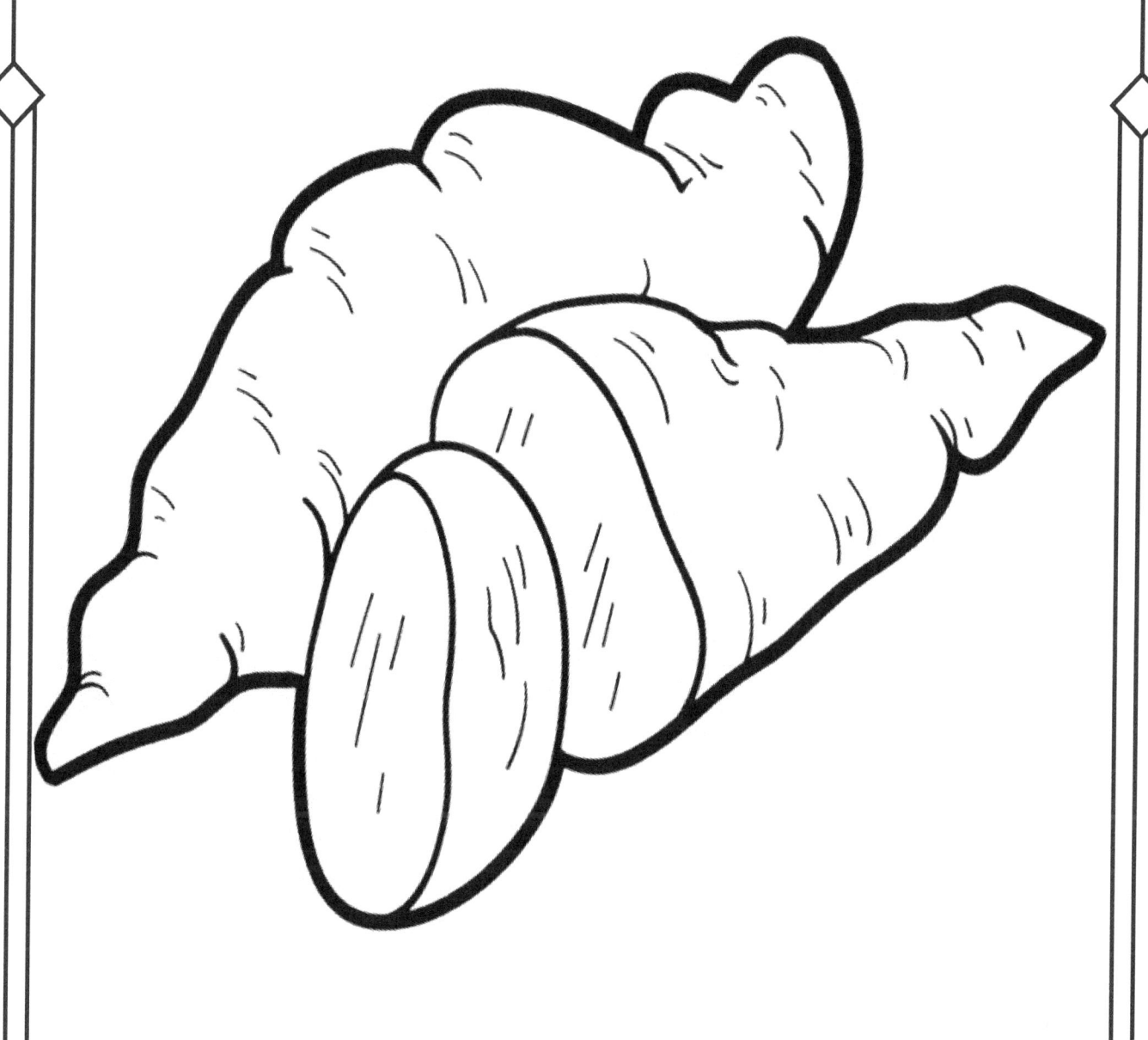

Sweet potato

Sweet potatoes are good for health because they are rich in fiber, vitamins, and antioxidants, supporting digestive health, boosting immunity, and promoting healthy skin.

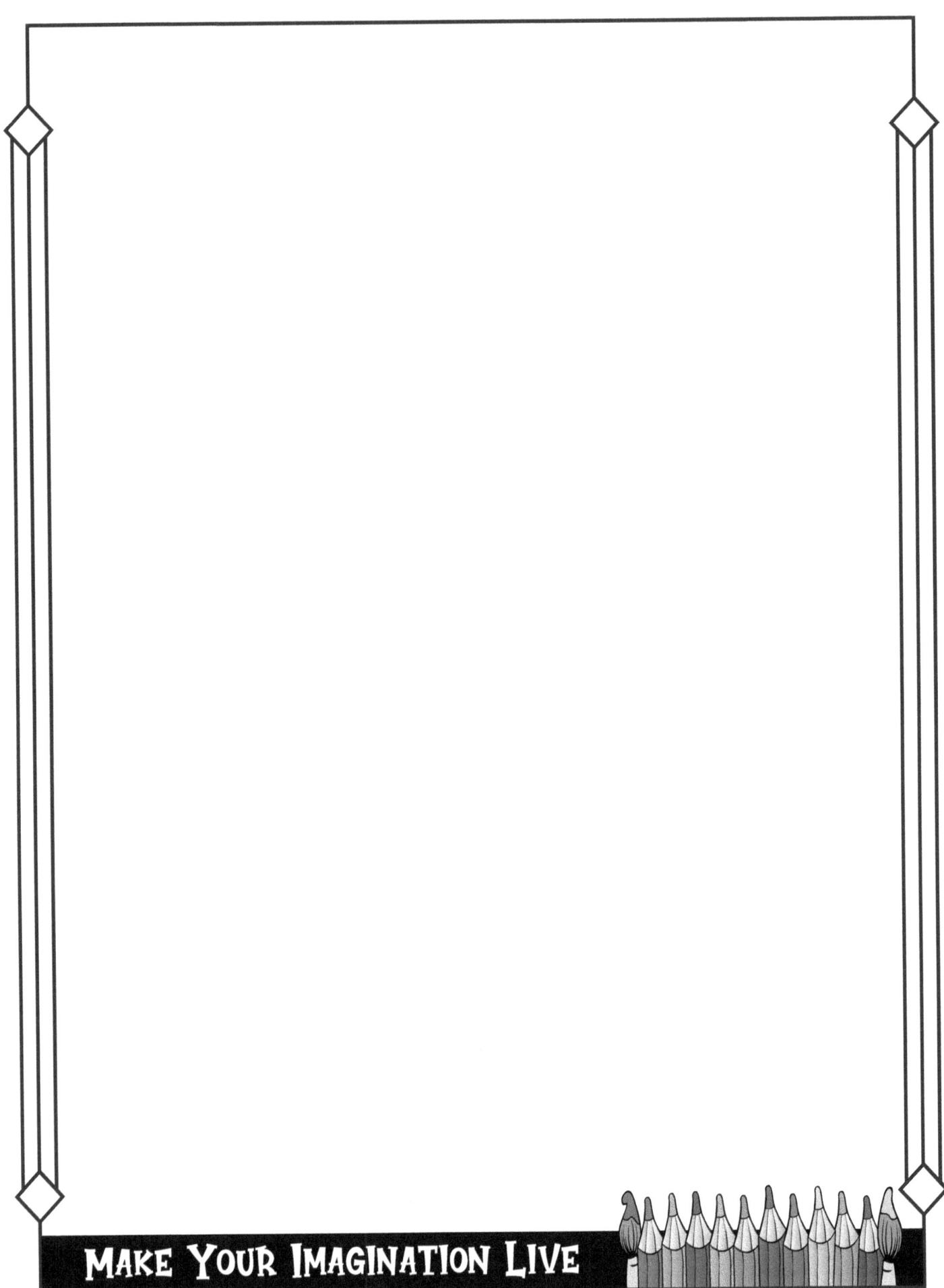

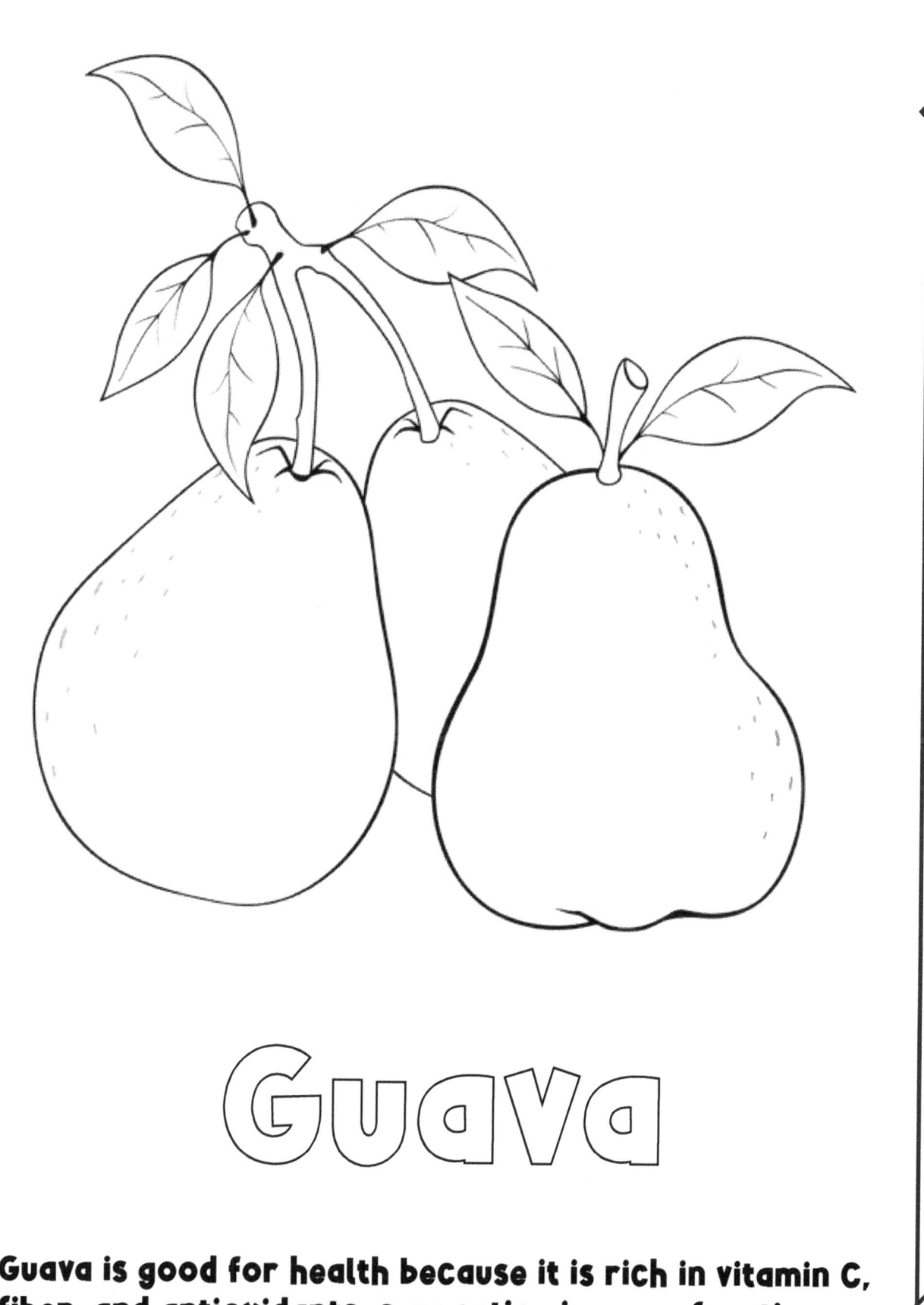

Guava

Guava is good for health because it is rich in vitamin C, fiber, and antioxidants, supporting immune function, digestion, and heart health.

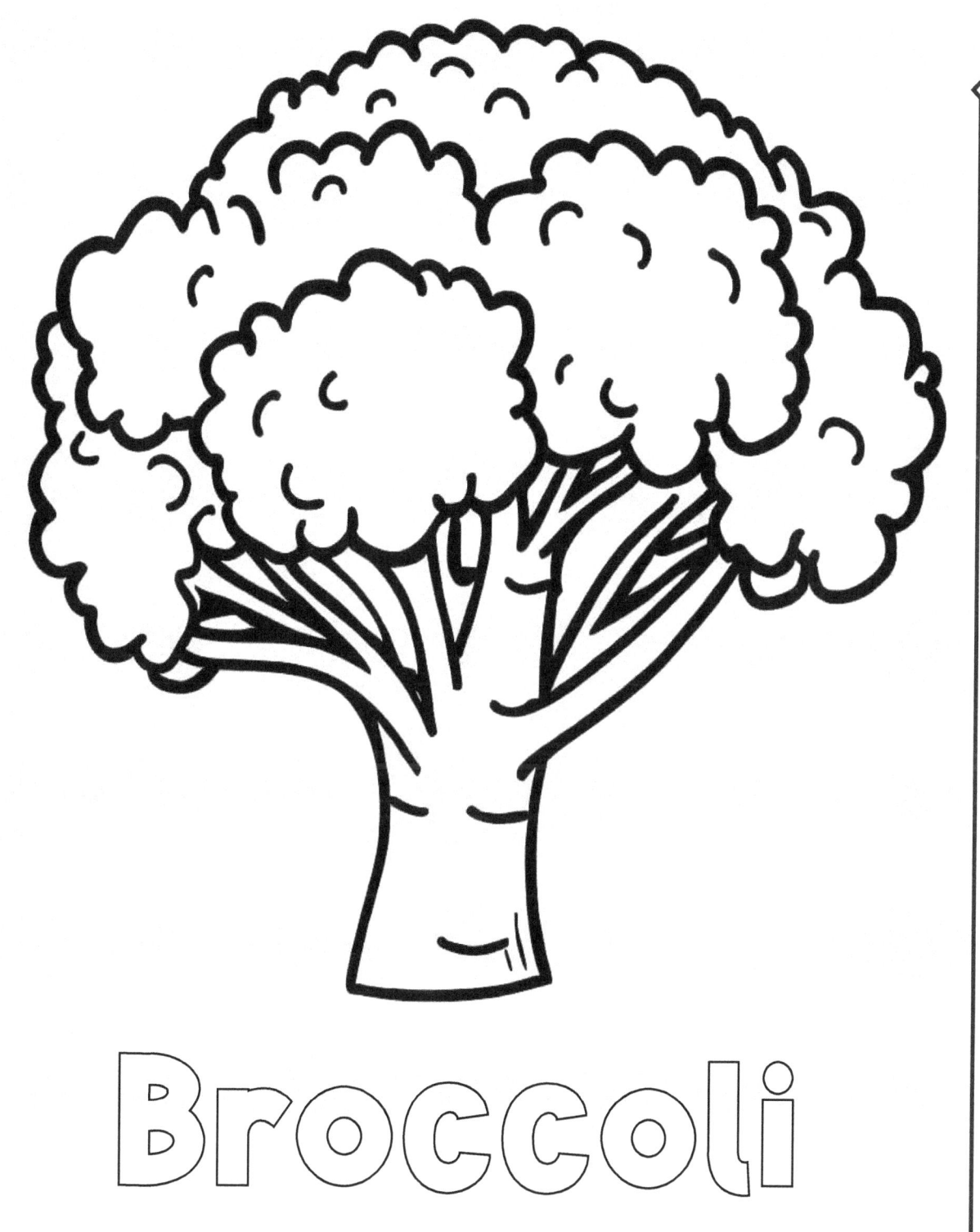

Broccoli

Broccoli is good for health because it is rich in vitamins, minerals, and antioxidants, supporting immune function, aiding digestion, and promoting heart health.

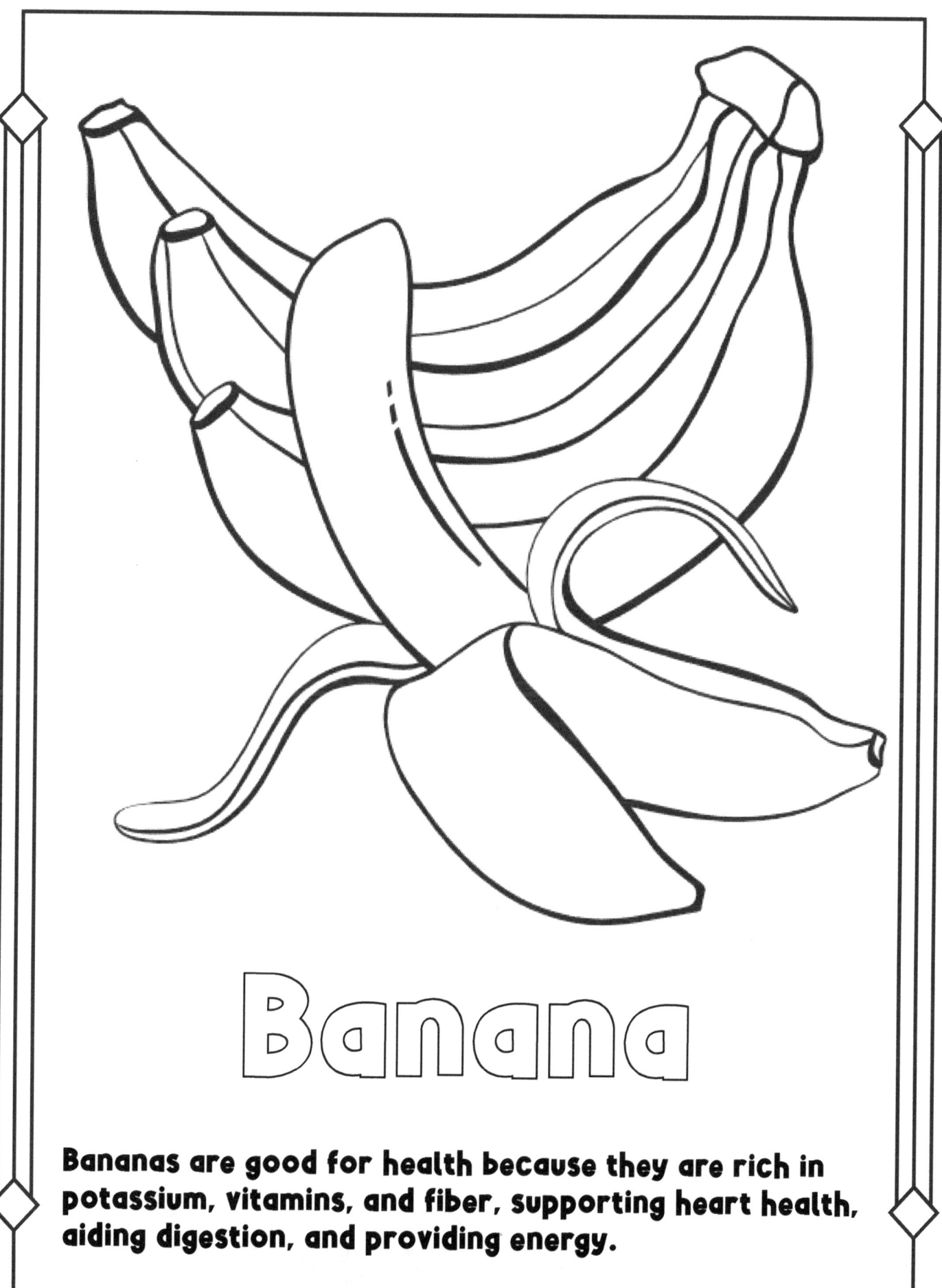

Banana

Bananas are good for health because they are rich in potassium, vitamins, and fiber, supporting heart health, aiding digestion, and providing energy.

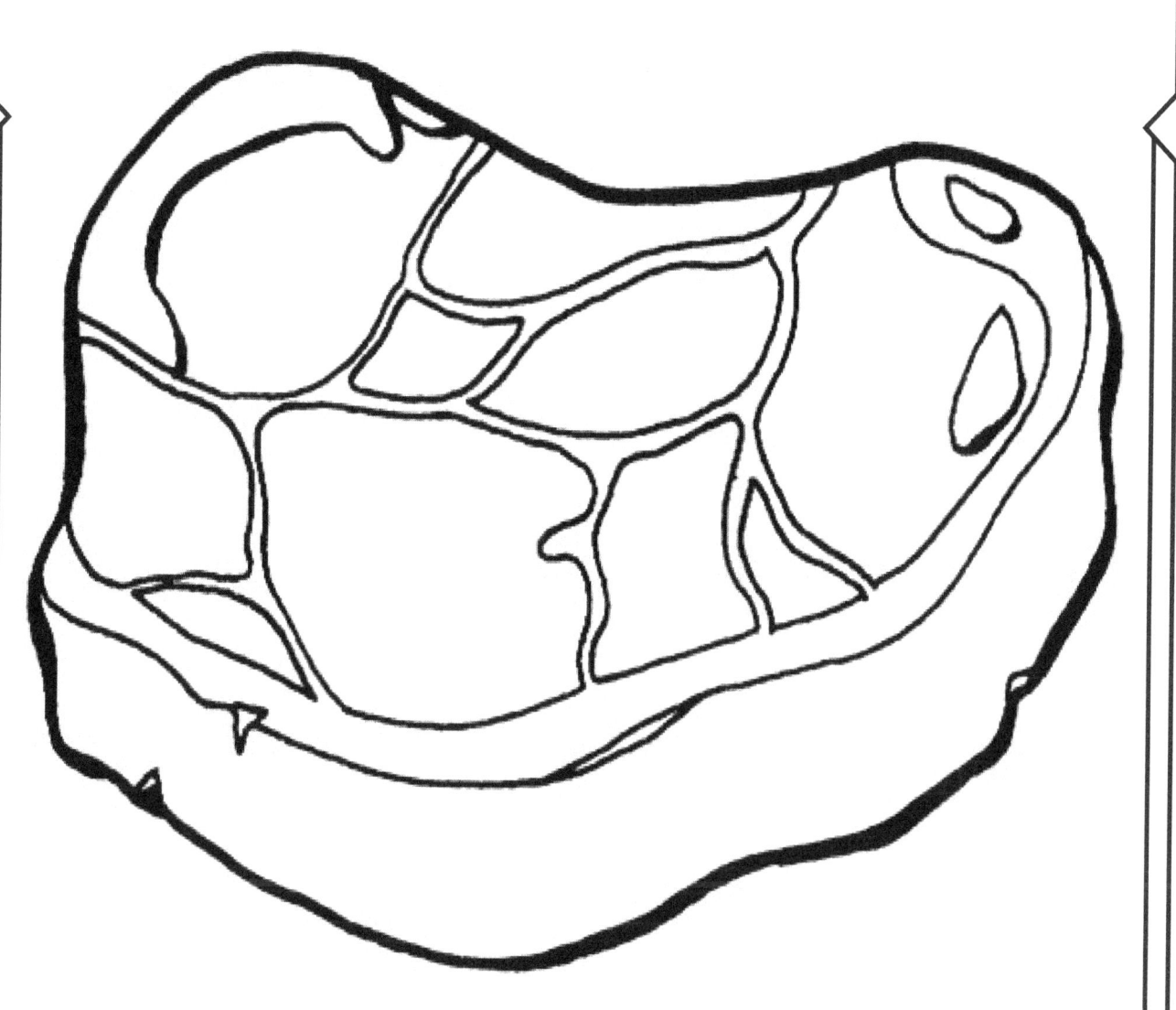

Lean Cuts Of Beef

Lean cuts of beef are good for health because they provide high-quality protein, iron, and essential nutrients with less saturated fat, supporting muscle growth, energy levels, and overall health.

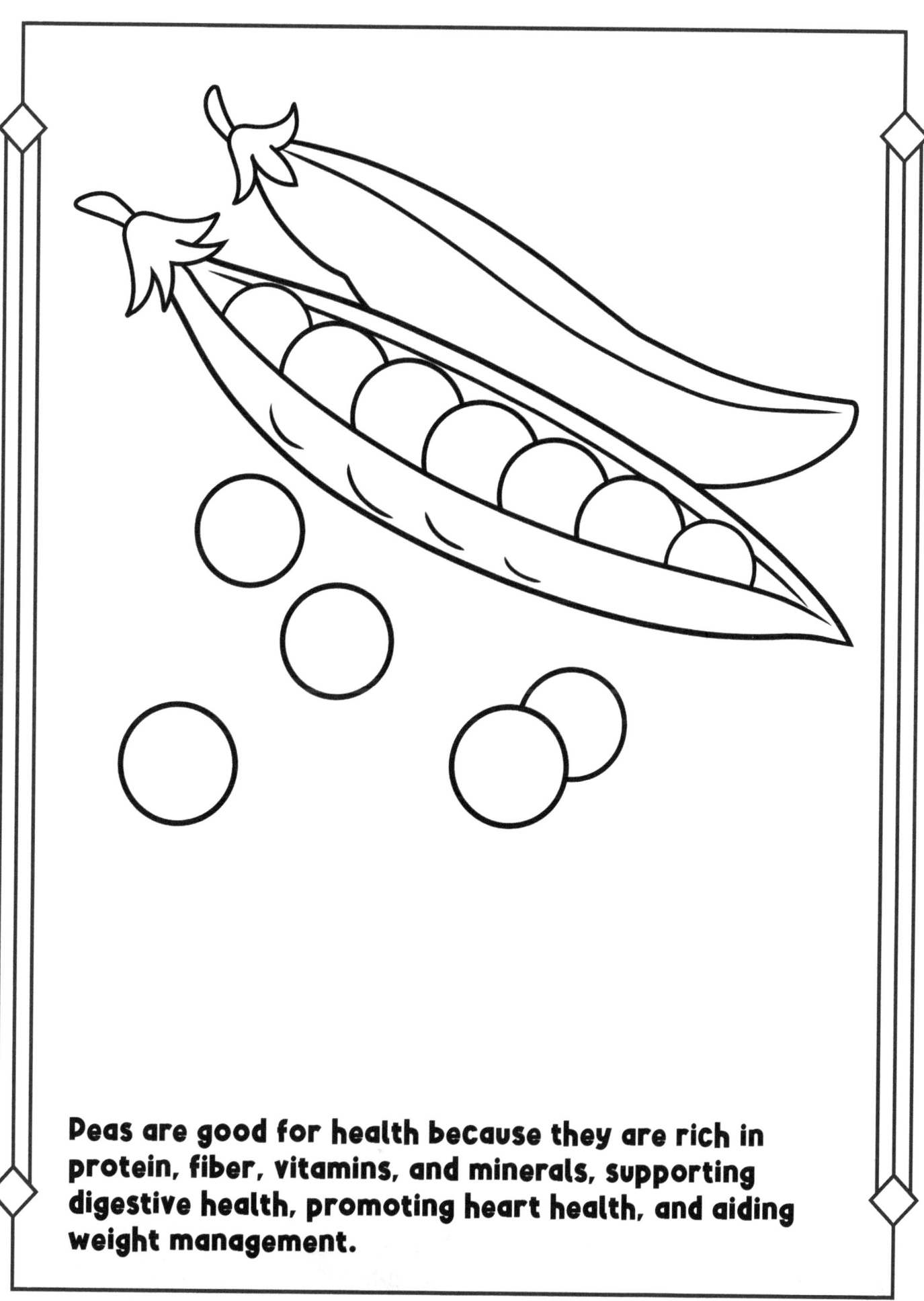

Peas are good for health because they are rich in protein, fiber, vitamins, and minerals, supporting digestive health, promoting heart health, and aiding weight management.

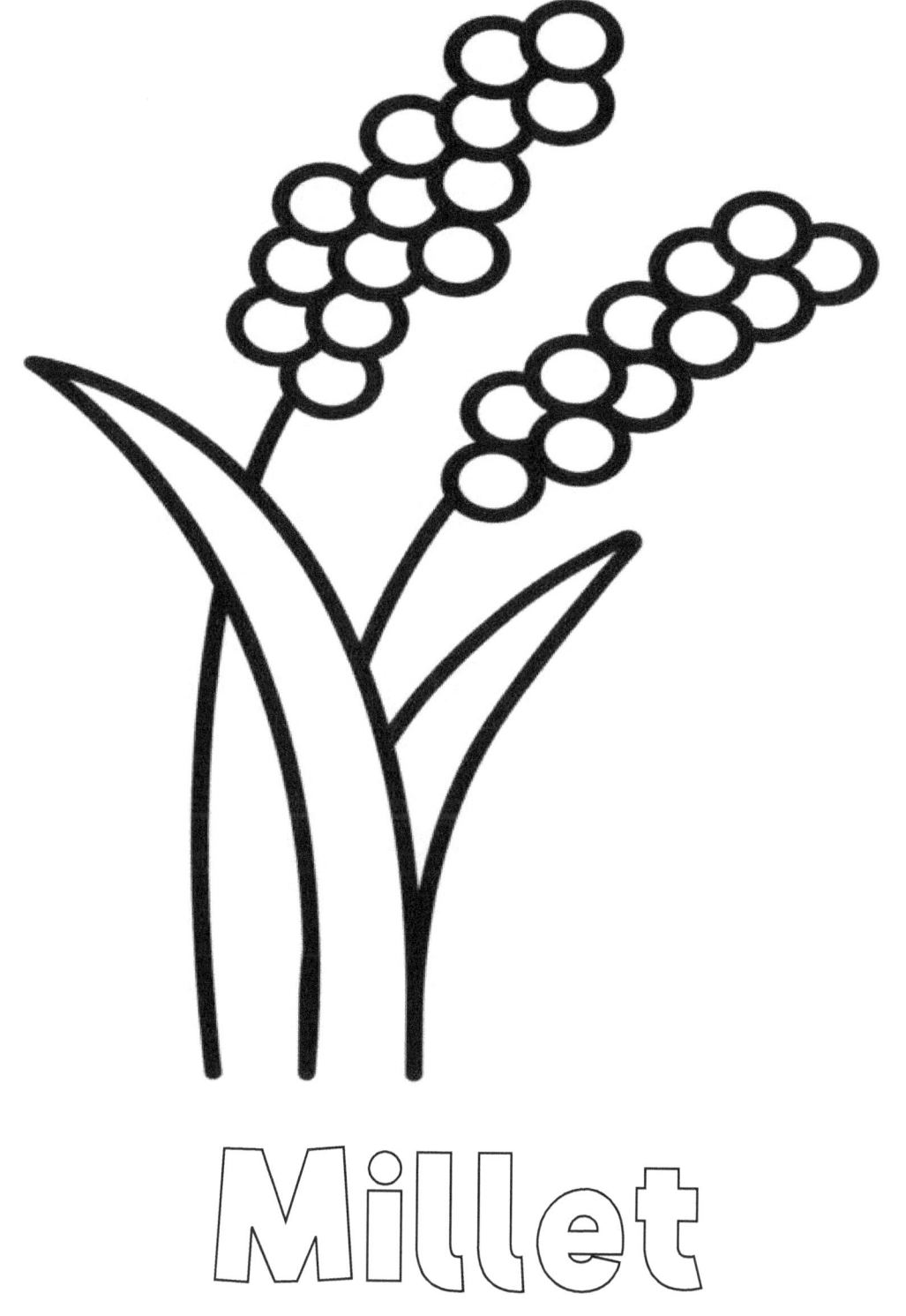

Millet

Millet is good for health because it is a gluten-free whole grain rich in nutrients, fiber, and antioxidants, supporting digestion, heart health, and blood sugar control.

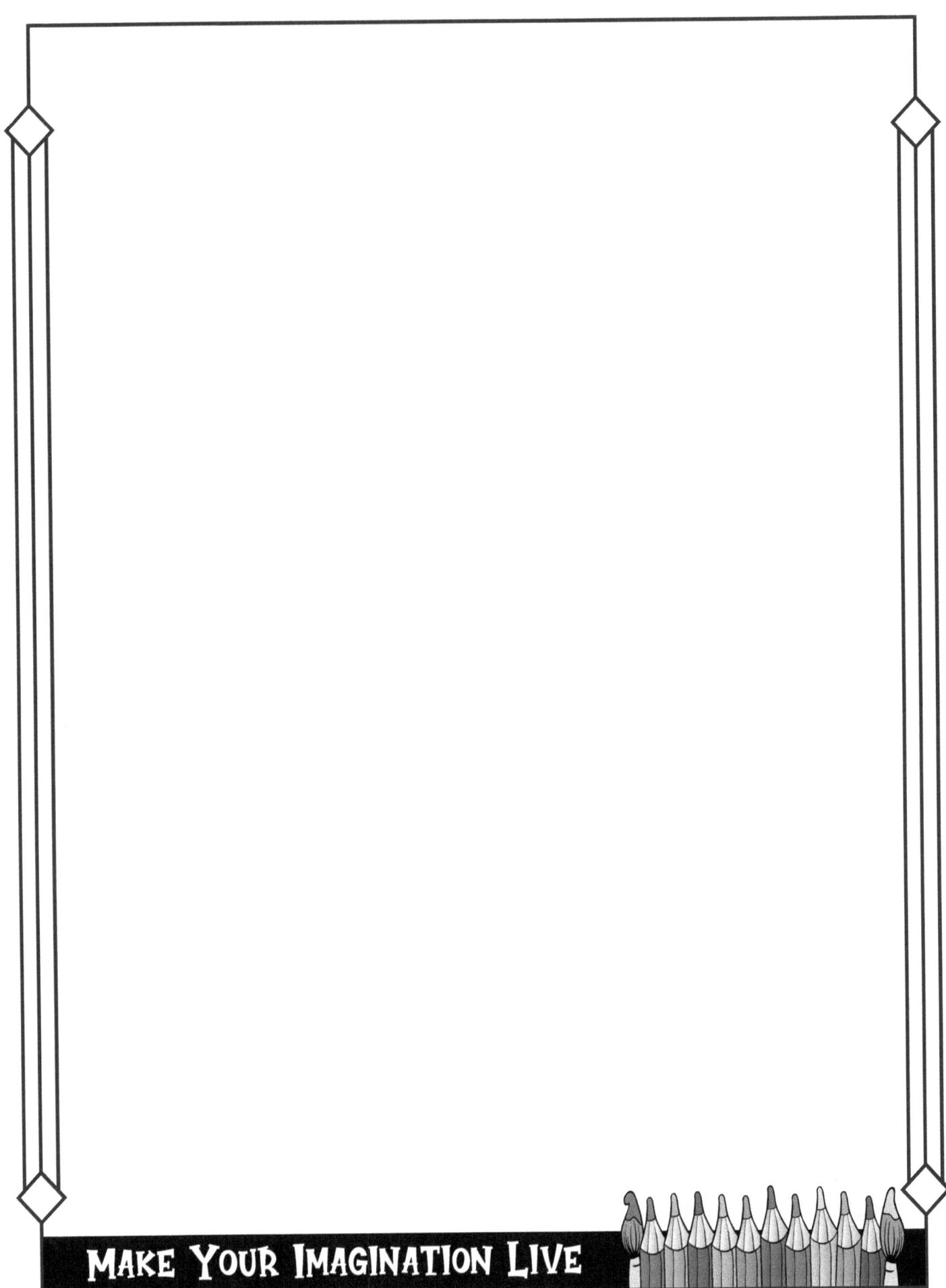

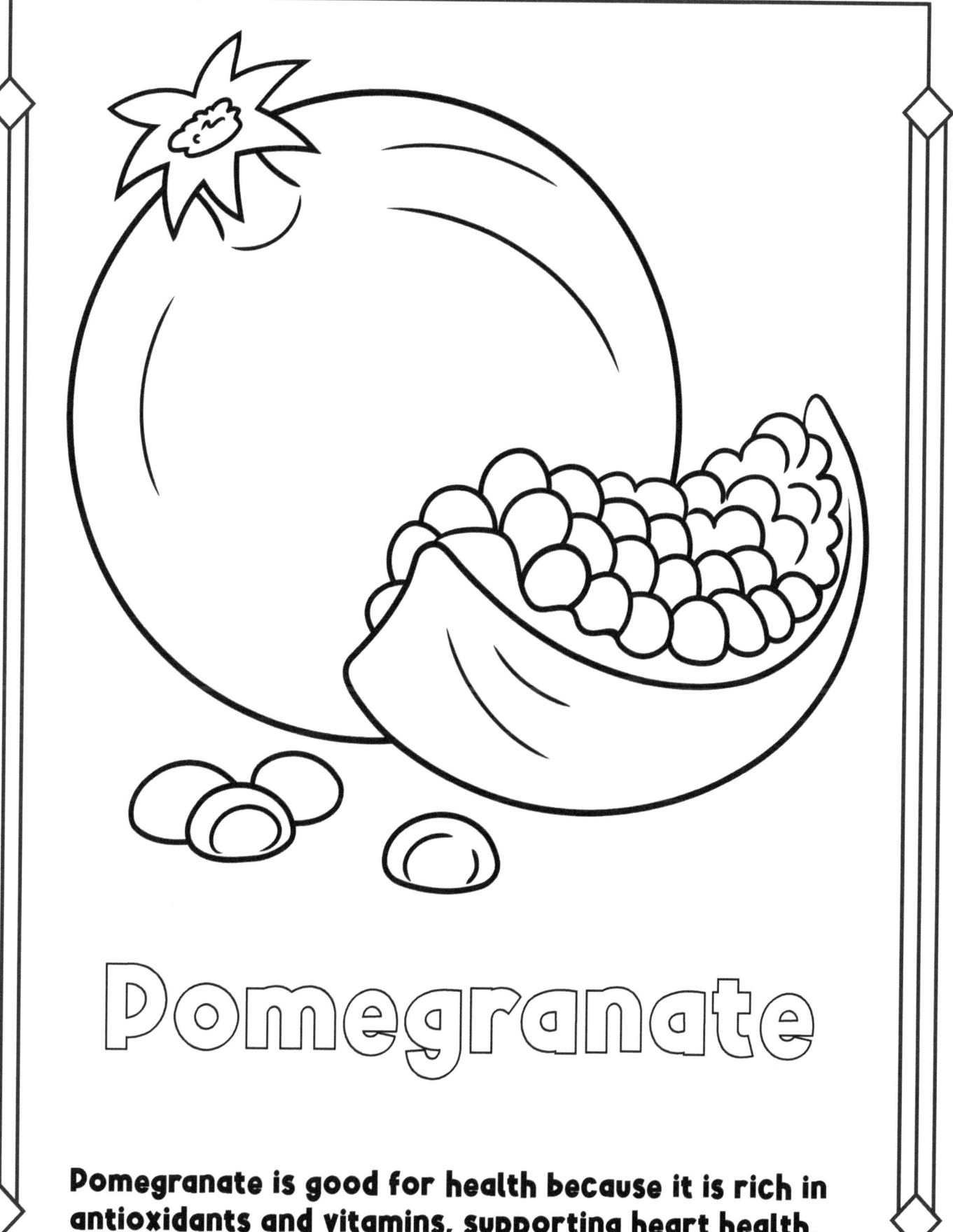

Pomegranate

Pomegranate is good for health because it is rich in antioxidants and vitamins, supporting heart health, reducing inflammation, and promoting healthy aging.

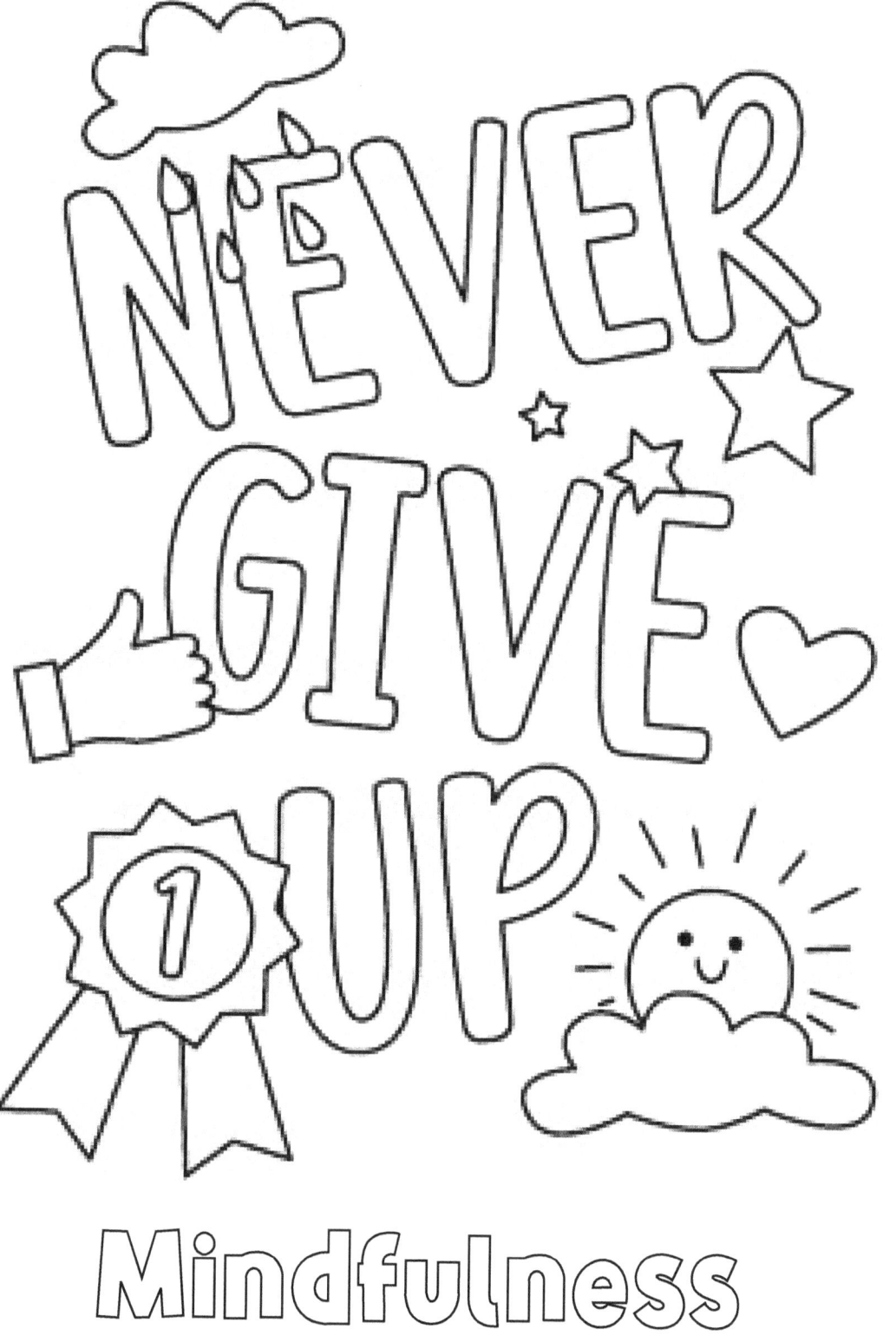

Mindfulness

Mindfulness is good for health because it reduces stress, enhances focus, promotes emotional well-being, and improves overall mental and physical health.

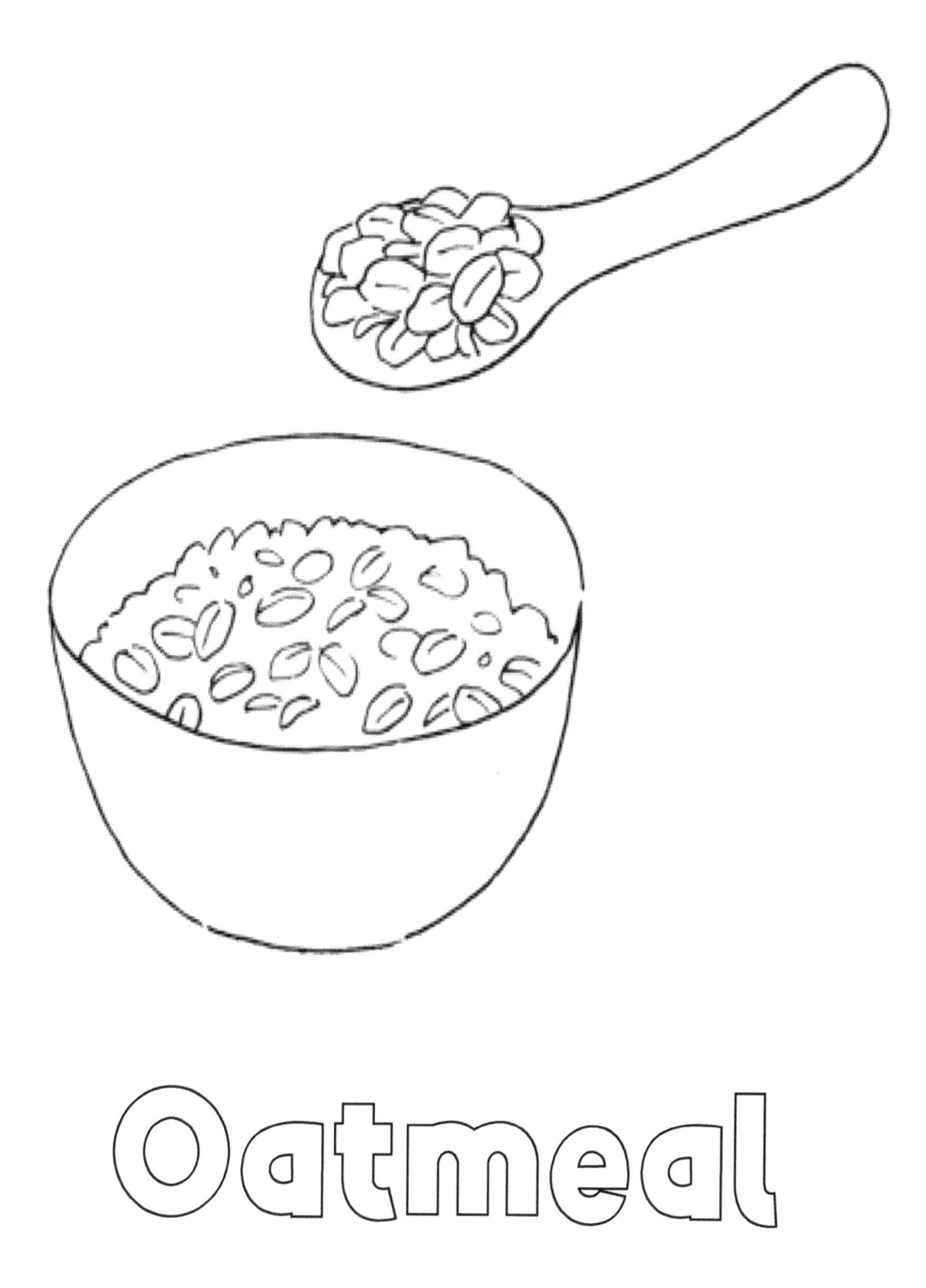

Oatmeal

Oatmeal is good for health because it is high in fiber, antioxidants, and nutrients, supporting heart health, digestion, and sustained energy levels.

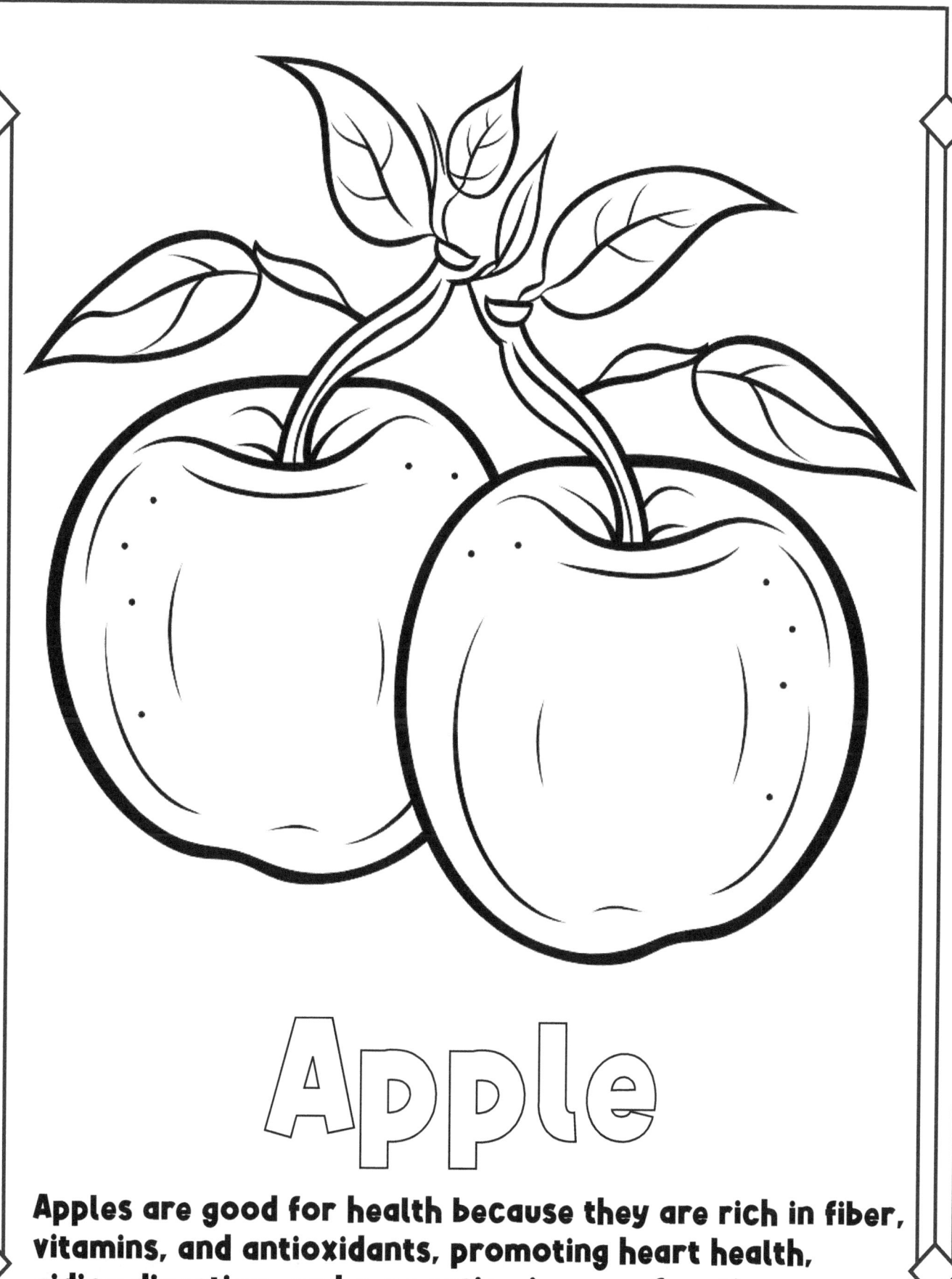

Apple

Apples are good for health because they are rich in fiber, vitamins, and antioxidants, promoting heart health, aiding digestion, and supporting immune function.

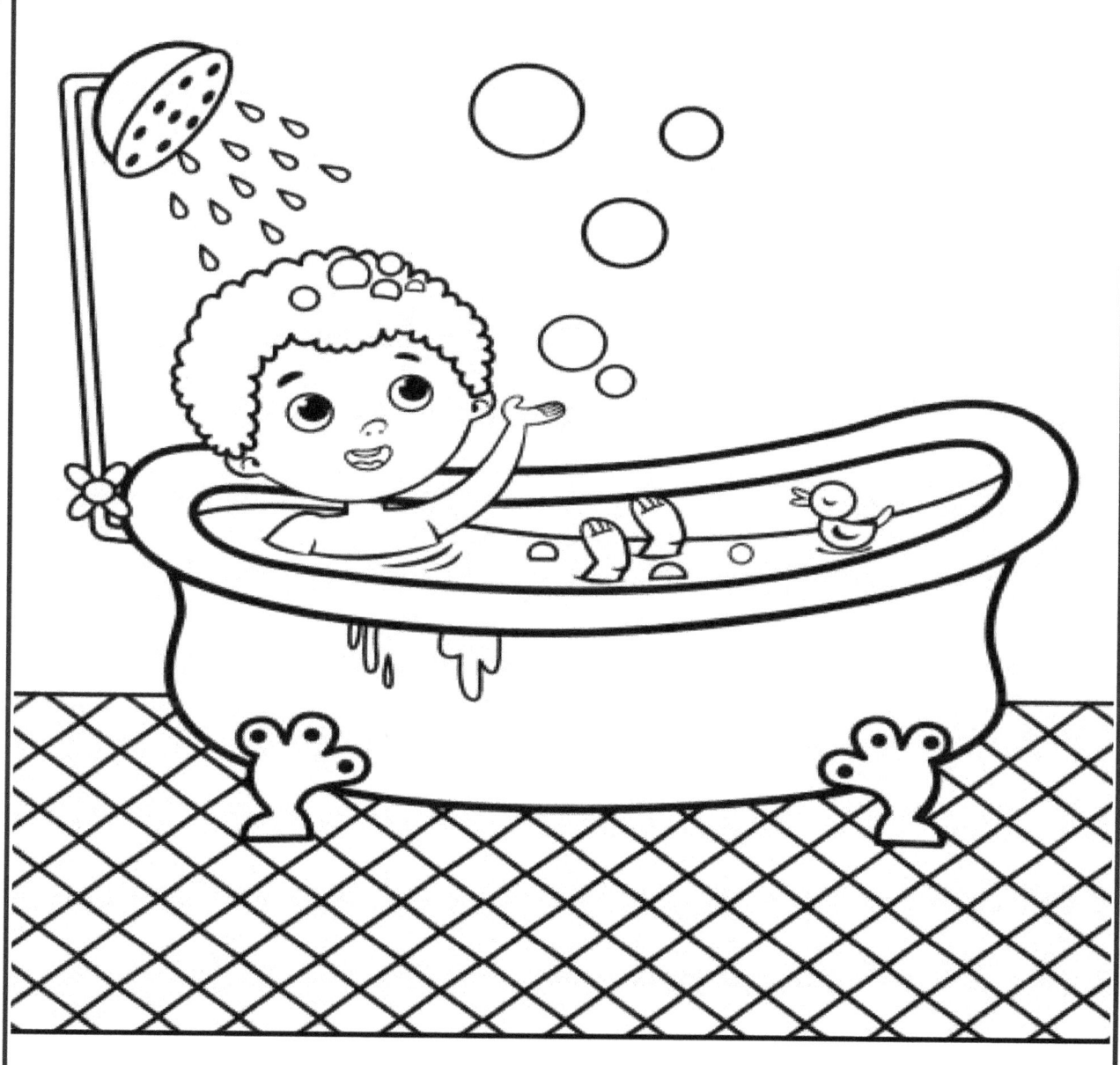

Practicing Good Hygiene

Practicing good hygiene is good for health because it helps prevent the spread of infections, reduces the risk of illness, and promotes overall well-being.

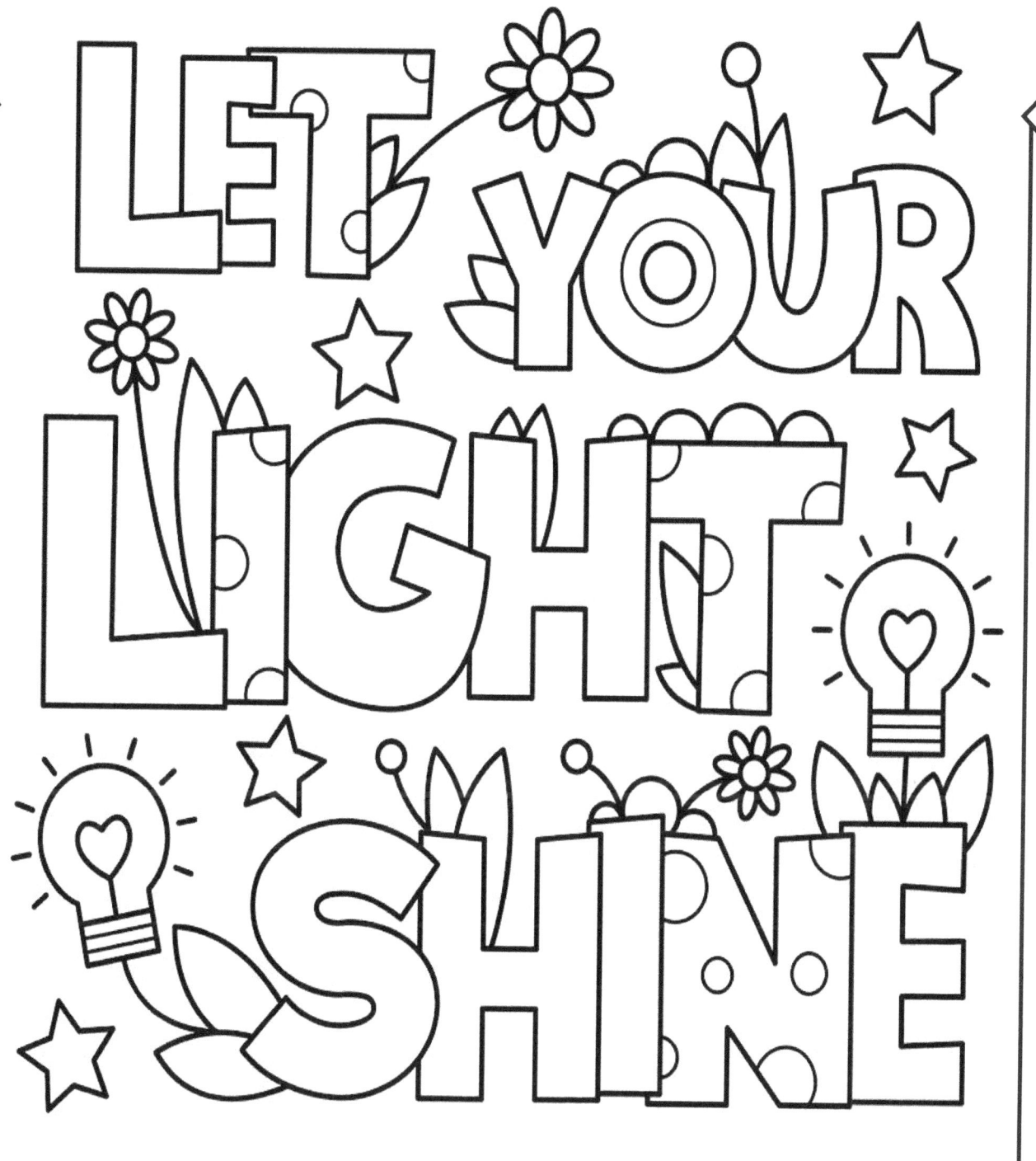

Reducing stress is good for health because it lowers the risk of chronic diseases, improves mental well-being, and enhances overall quality of life.

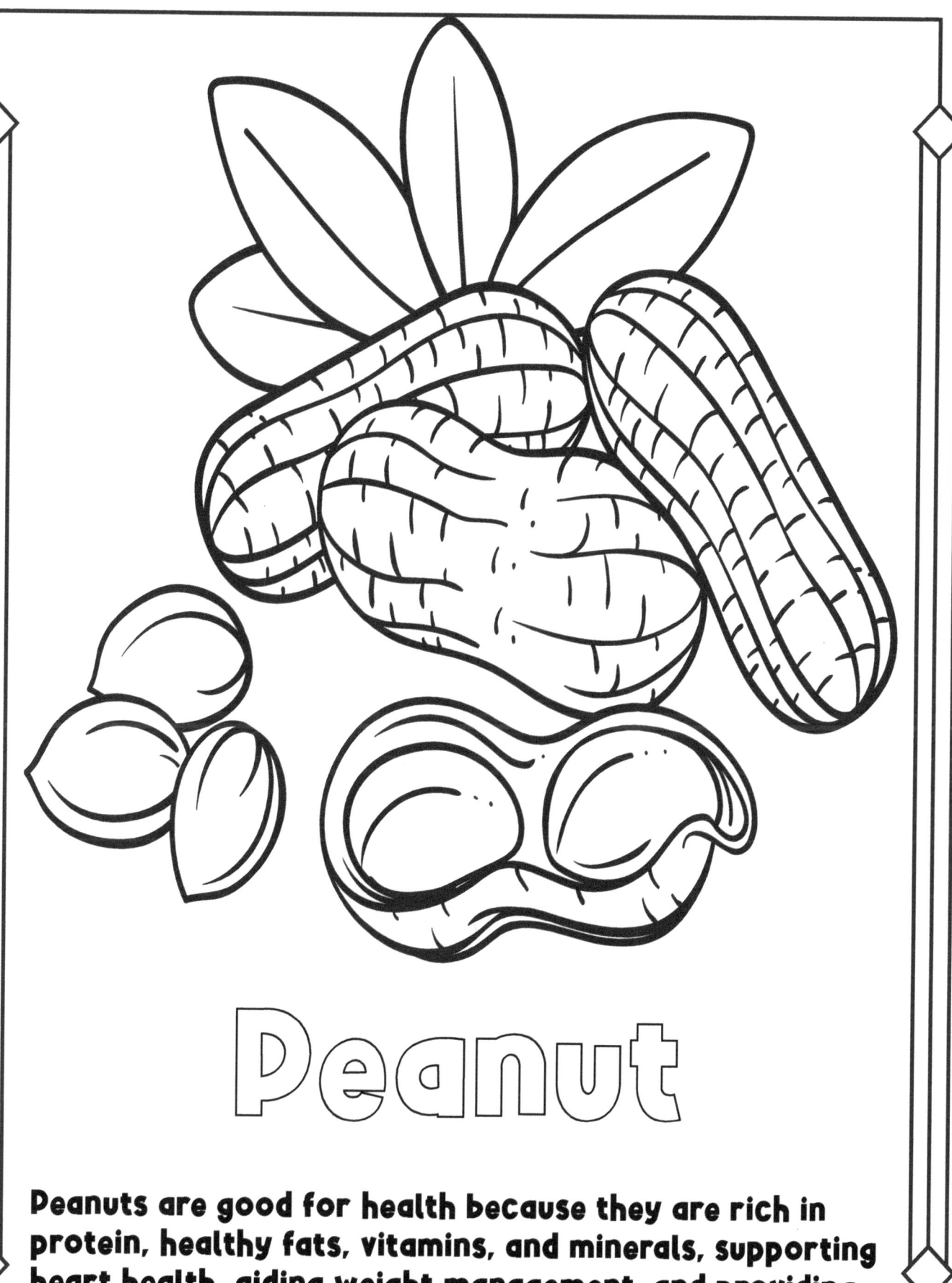

Peanut

Peanuts are good for health because they are rich in protein, healthy fats, vitamins, and minerals, supporting heart health, aiding weight management, and providing energy.

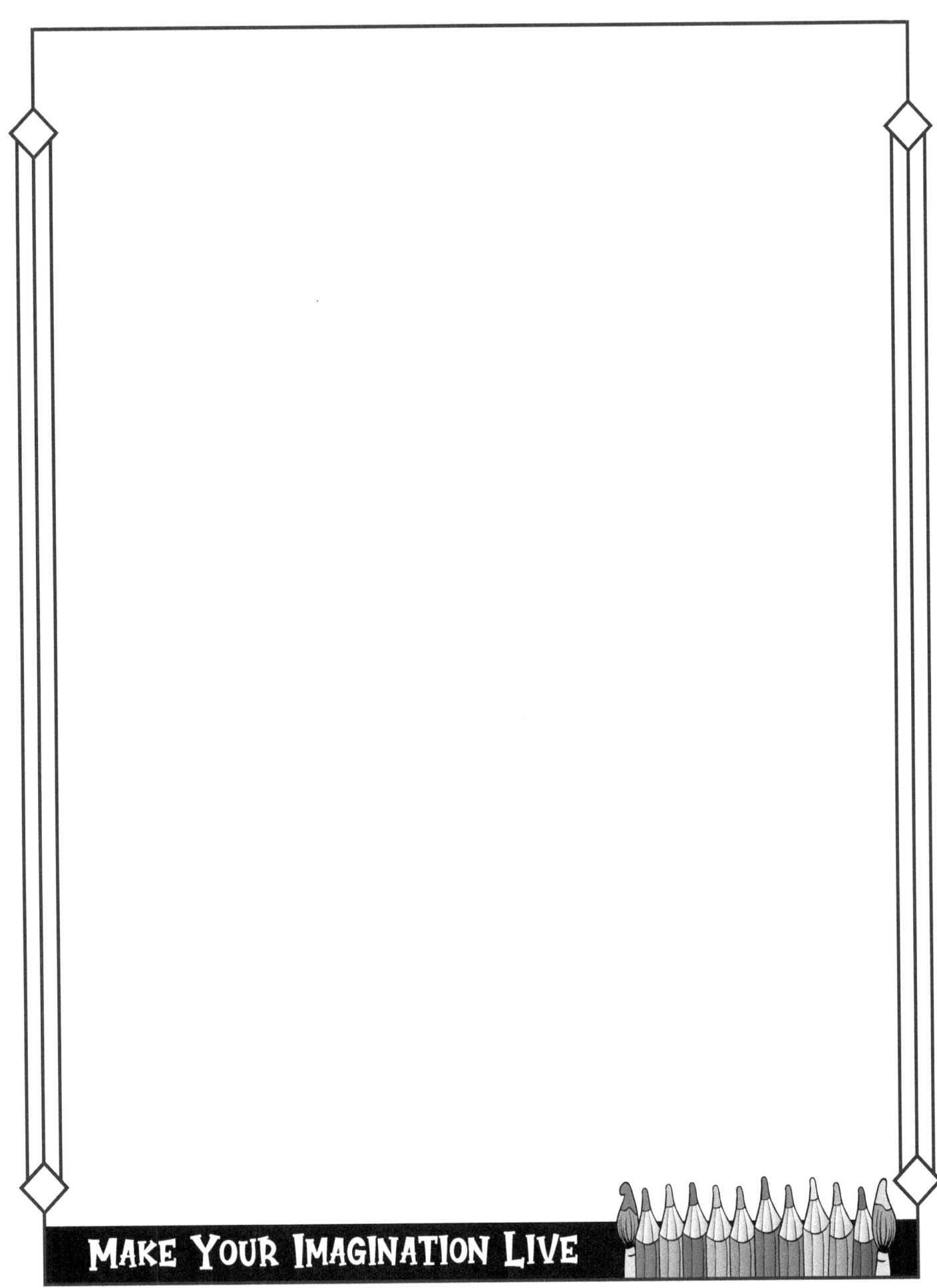

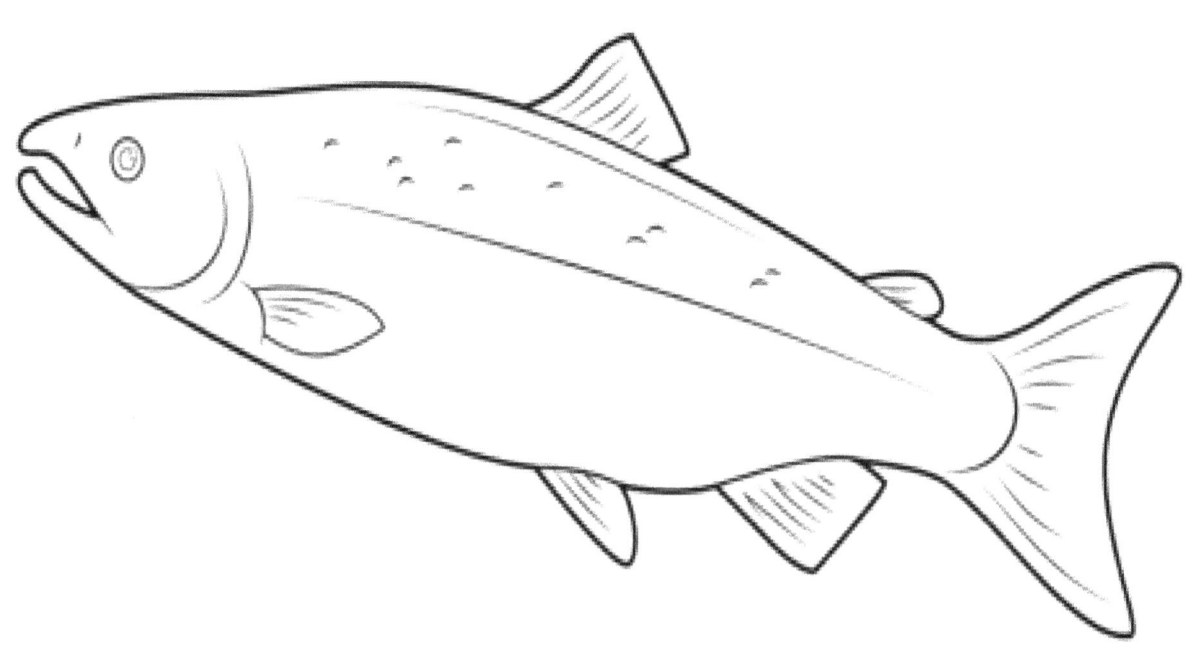

Salmon Fish

Salmon fish is good for health because it is rich in omega-3 fatty acids, protein, and essential nutrients, supporting heart health, brain function, and reducing inflammation.

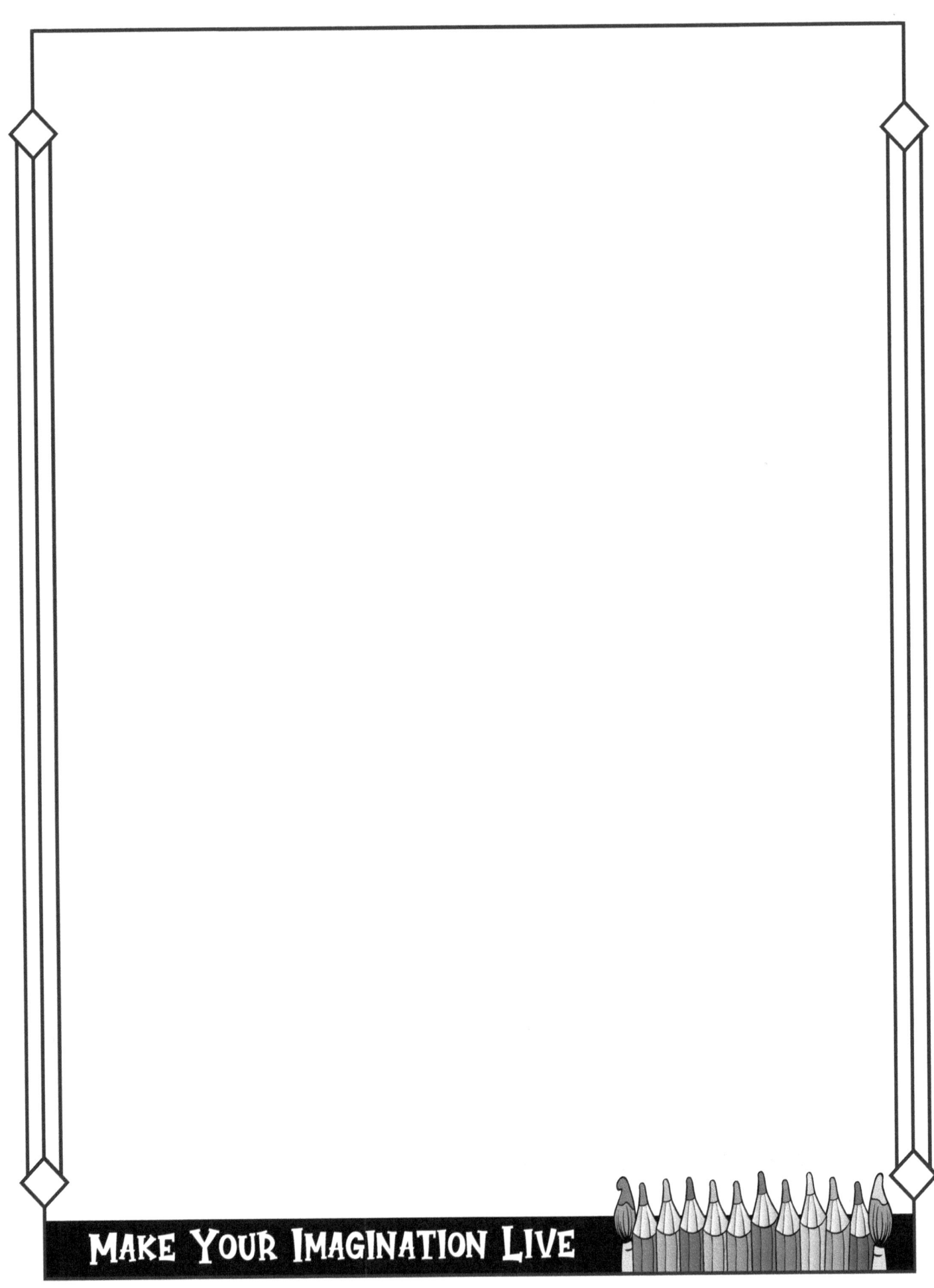

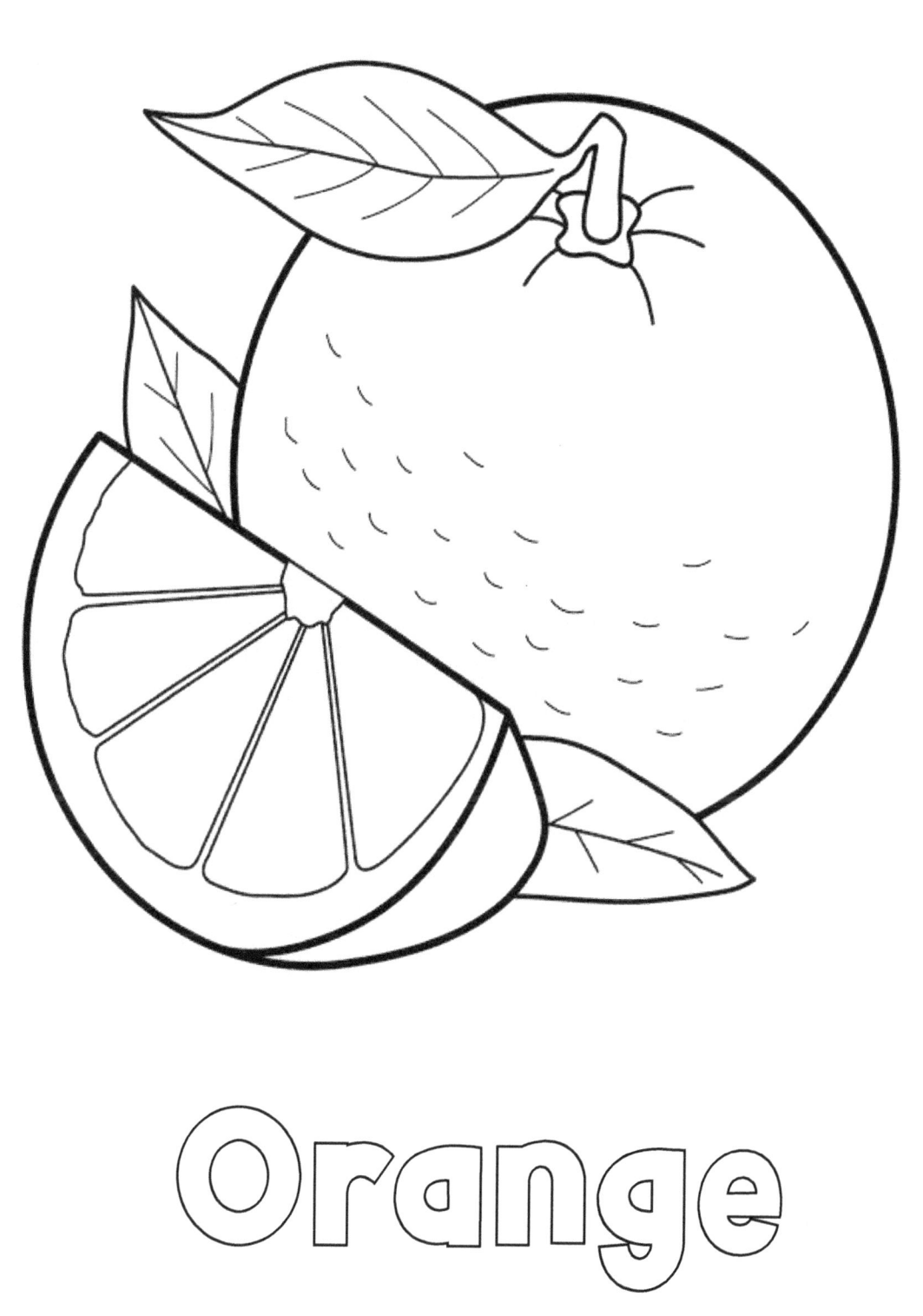

Orange

Oranges are good for health because they are rich in vitamin C, antioxidants, and fiber, supporting immune function, aiding digestion, and promoting heart health.

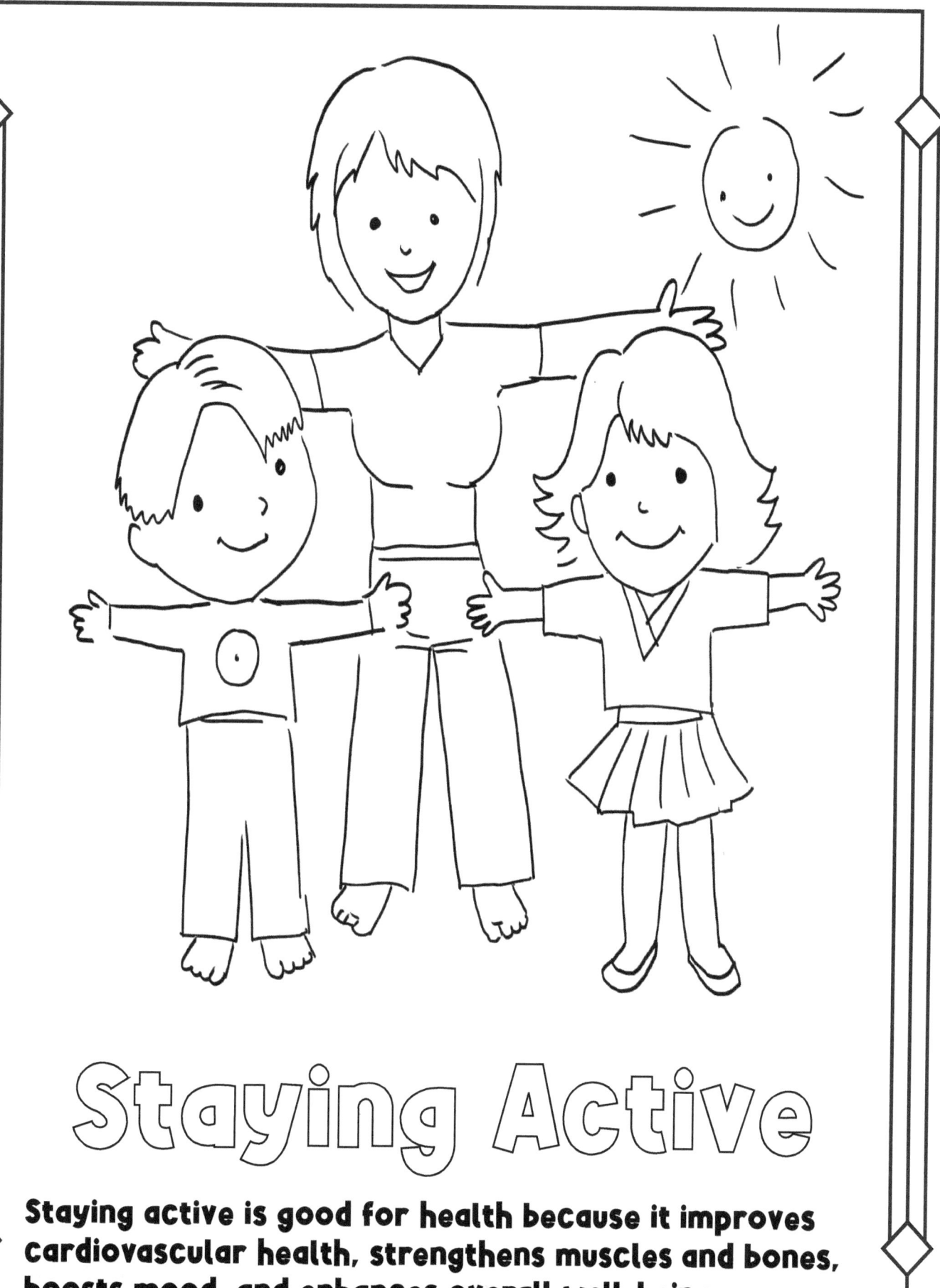

Staying Active

Staying active is good for health because it improves cardiovascular health, strengthens muscles and bones, boosts mood, and enhances overall well-being.

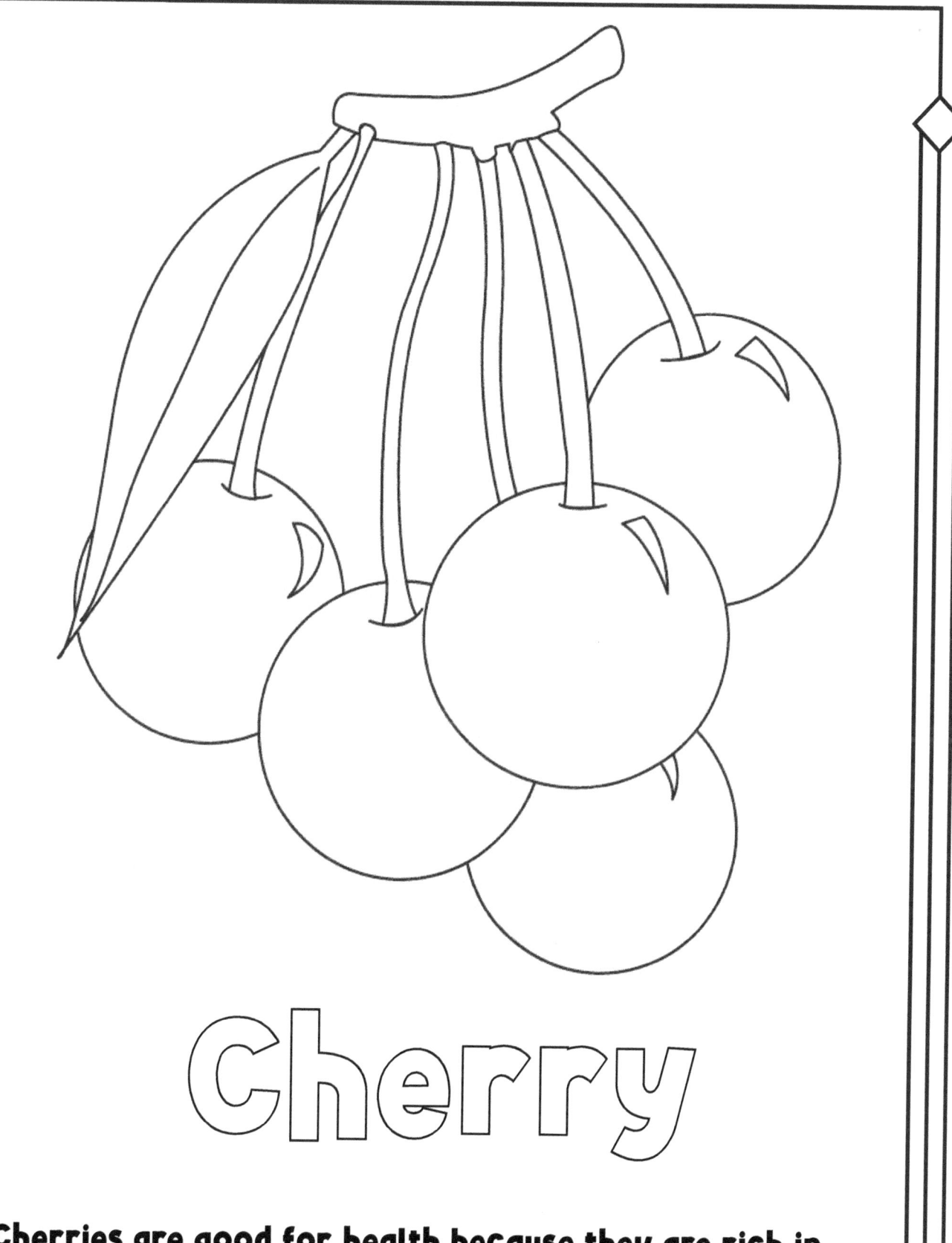

Cherry

Cherries are good for health because they are rich in antioxidants and anti-inflammatory compounds, supporting heart health, aiding sleep, and reducing muscle soreness.

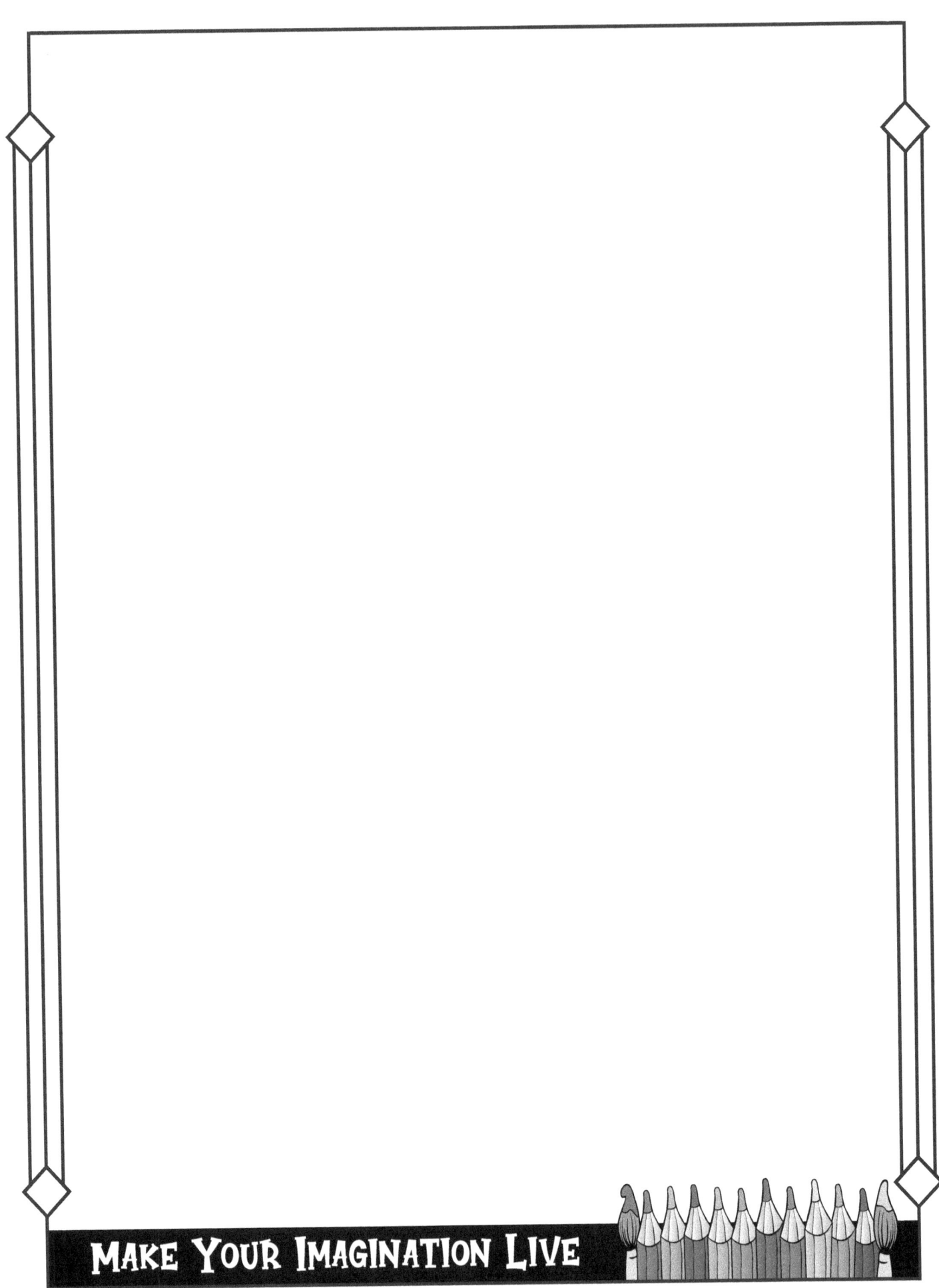

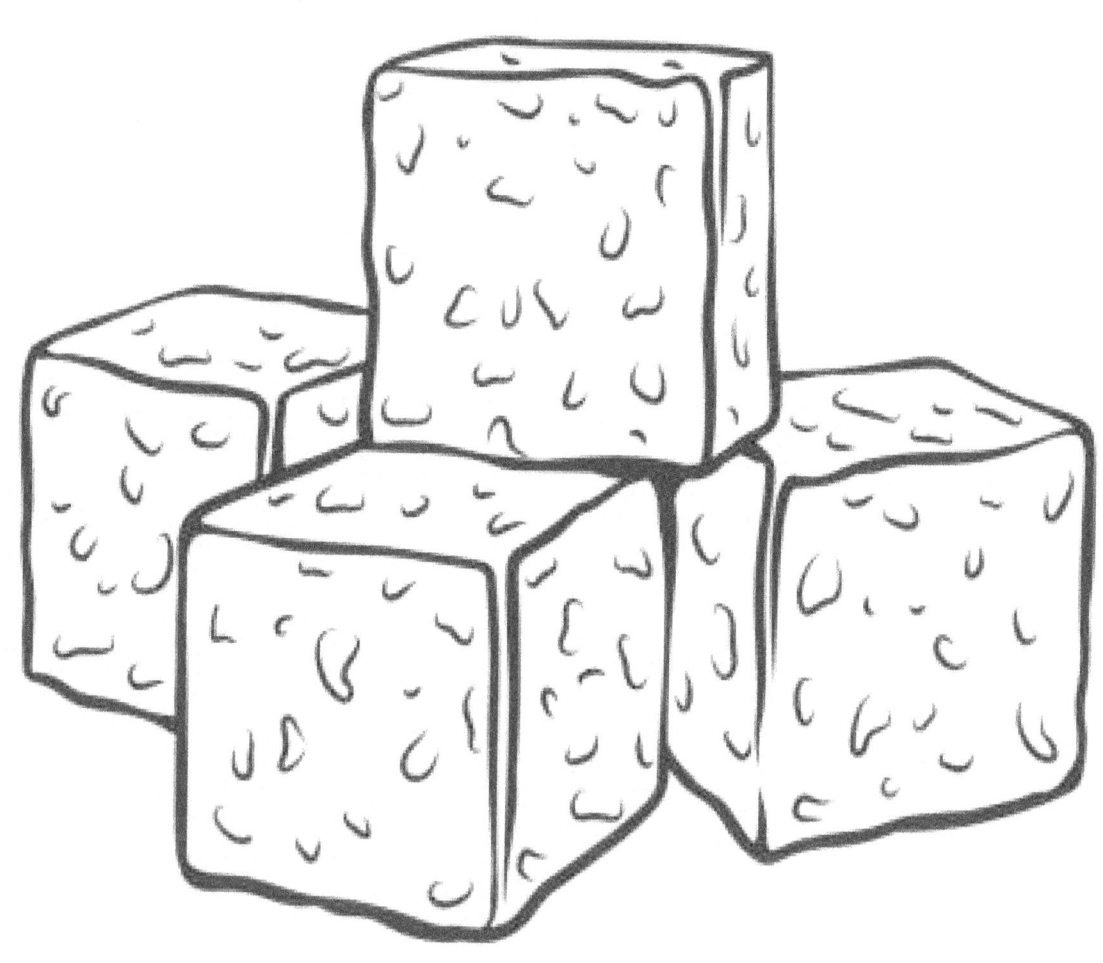

Tofu

Tofu also contains all the essential amino acids your body needs and is rich in minerals and vitamins, including calcium, manganese, iron and vitamin A.

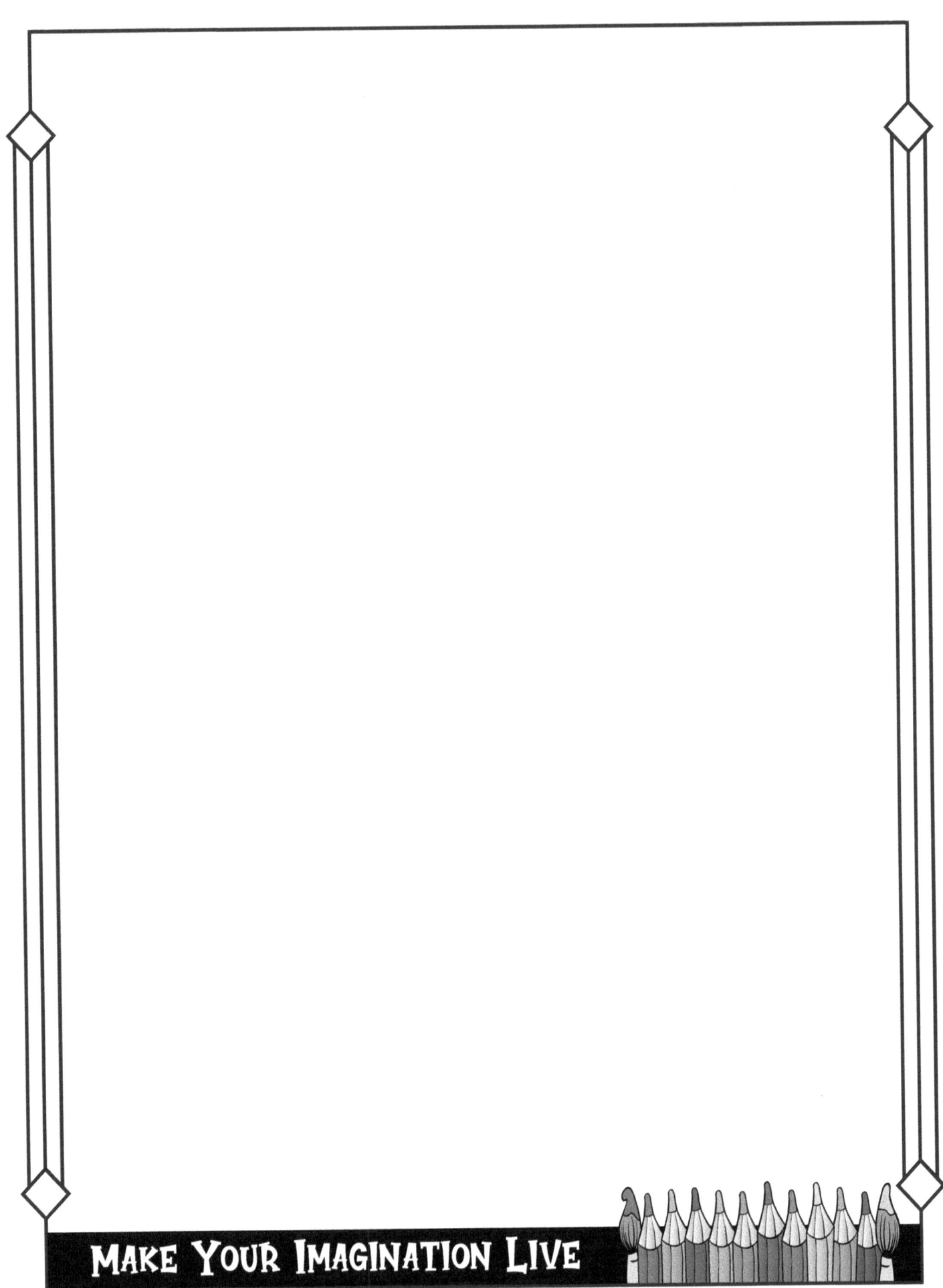

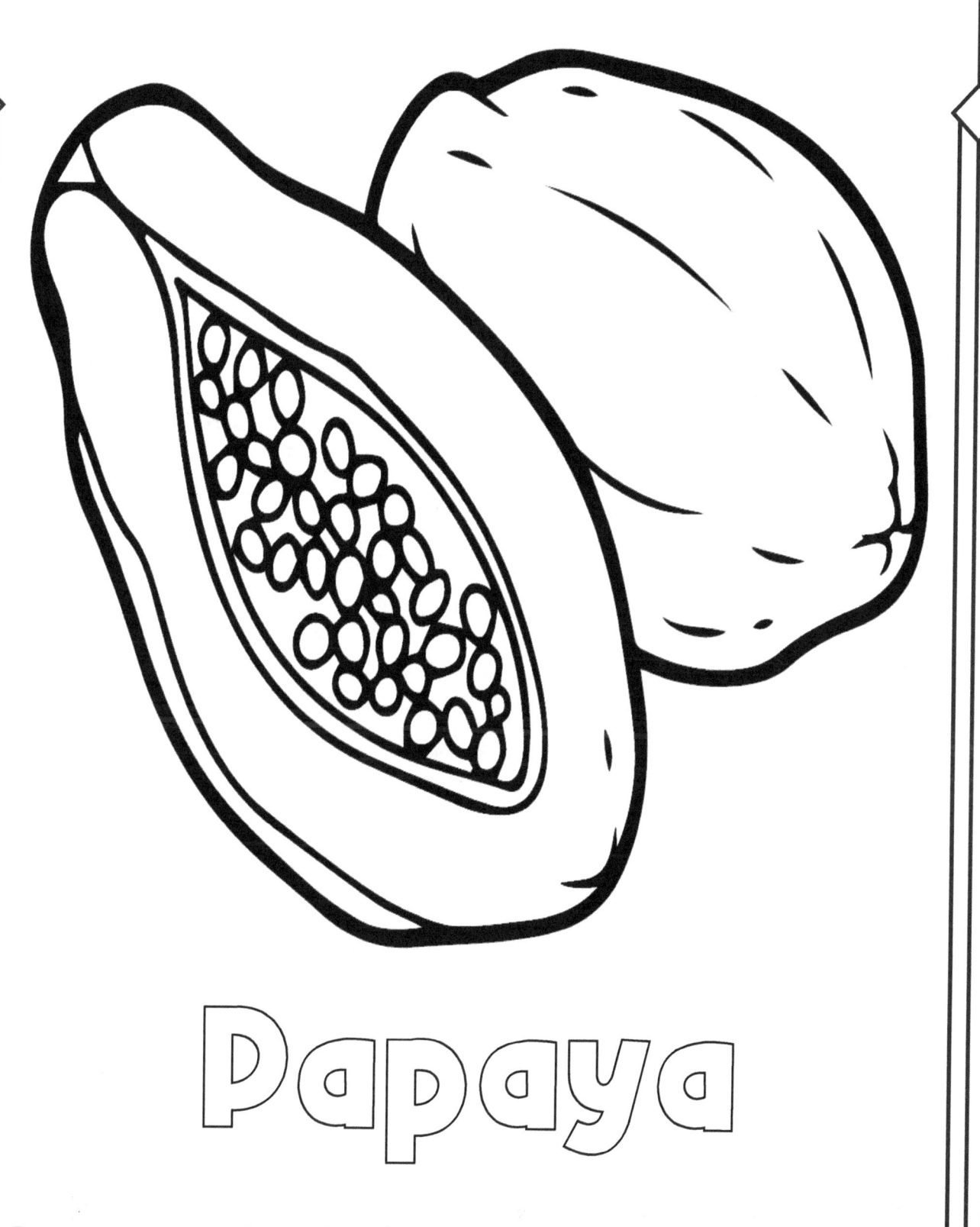

Papaya

Papaya is good for health because it is rich in vitamins, minerals, and antioxidants, aiding digestion, supporting immune function, and promoting skin health.

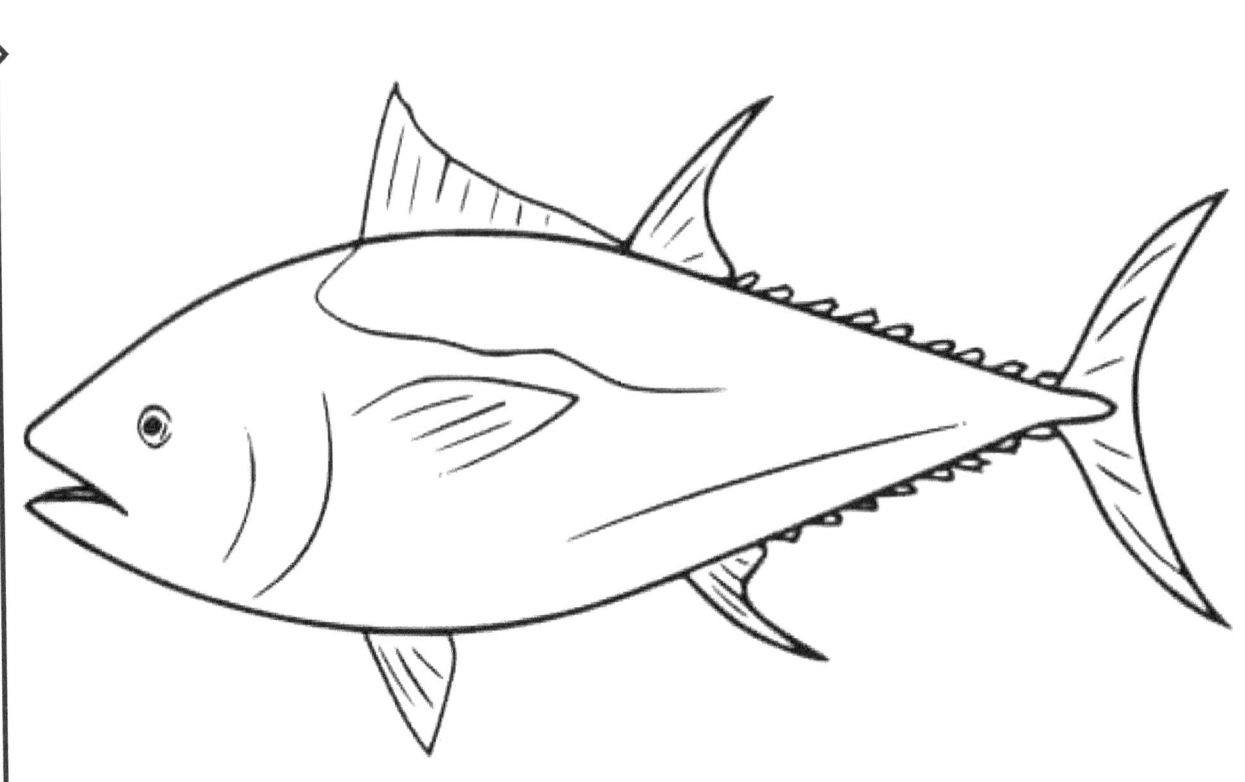

Tuna Fish

Tuna is a lean meat. It's relatively high in protein, but low in calories, which means that it keeps you full longer and stops you from eating more

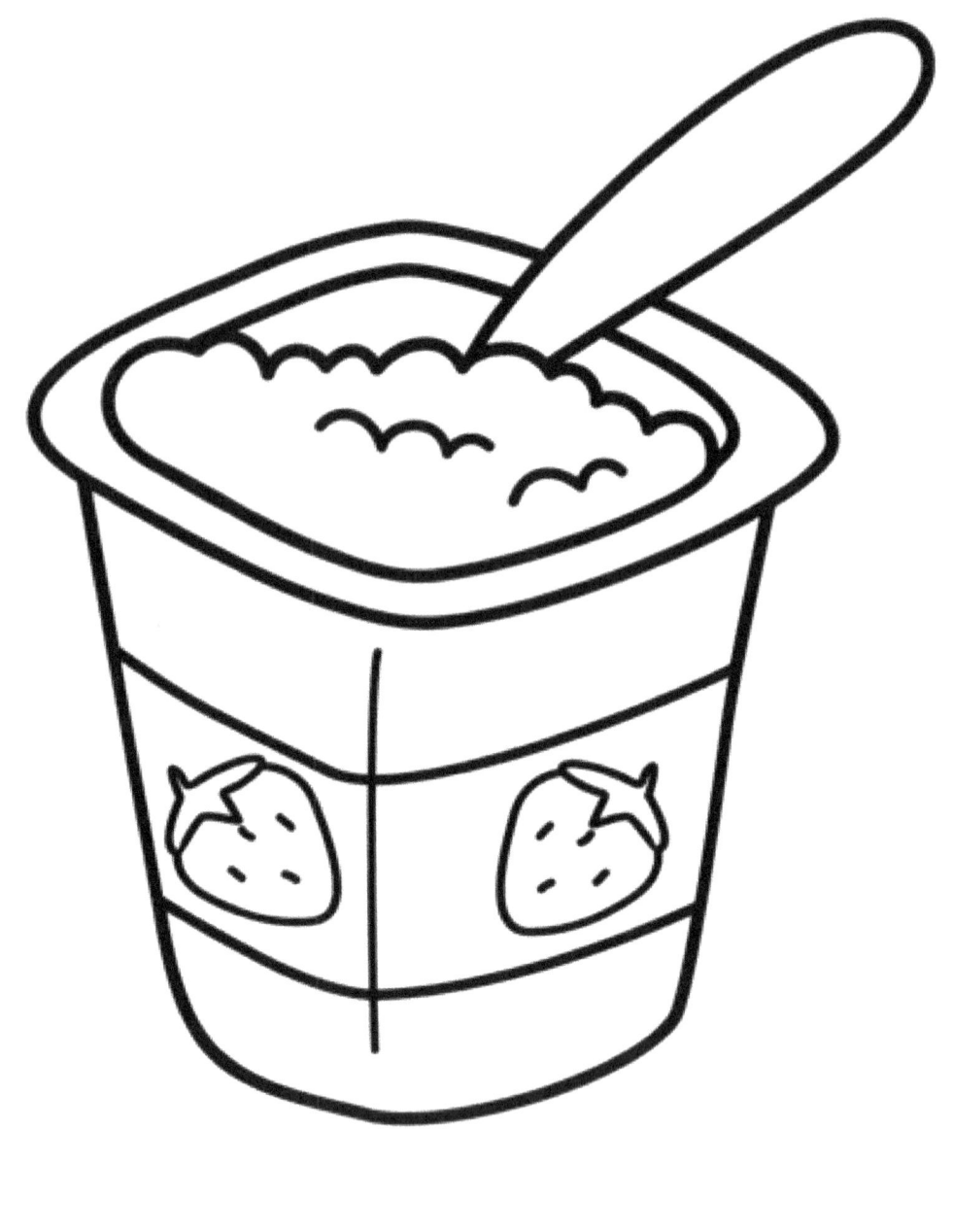

Yogurt

Yogurts can be high in protein, calcium, vitamins, and live culture, or probiotics, which can enhance the gut microbiota.

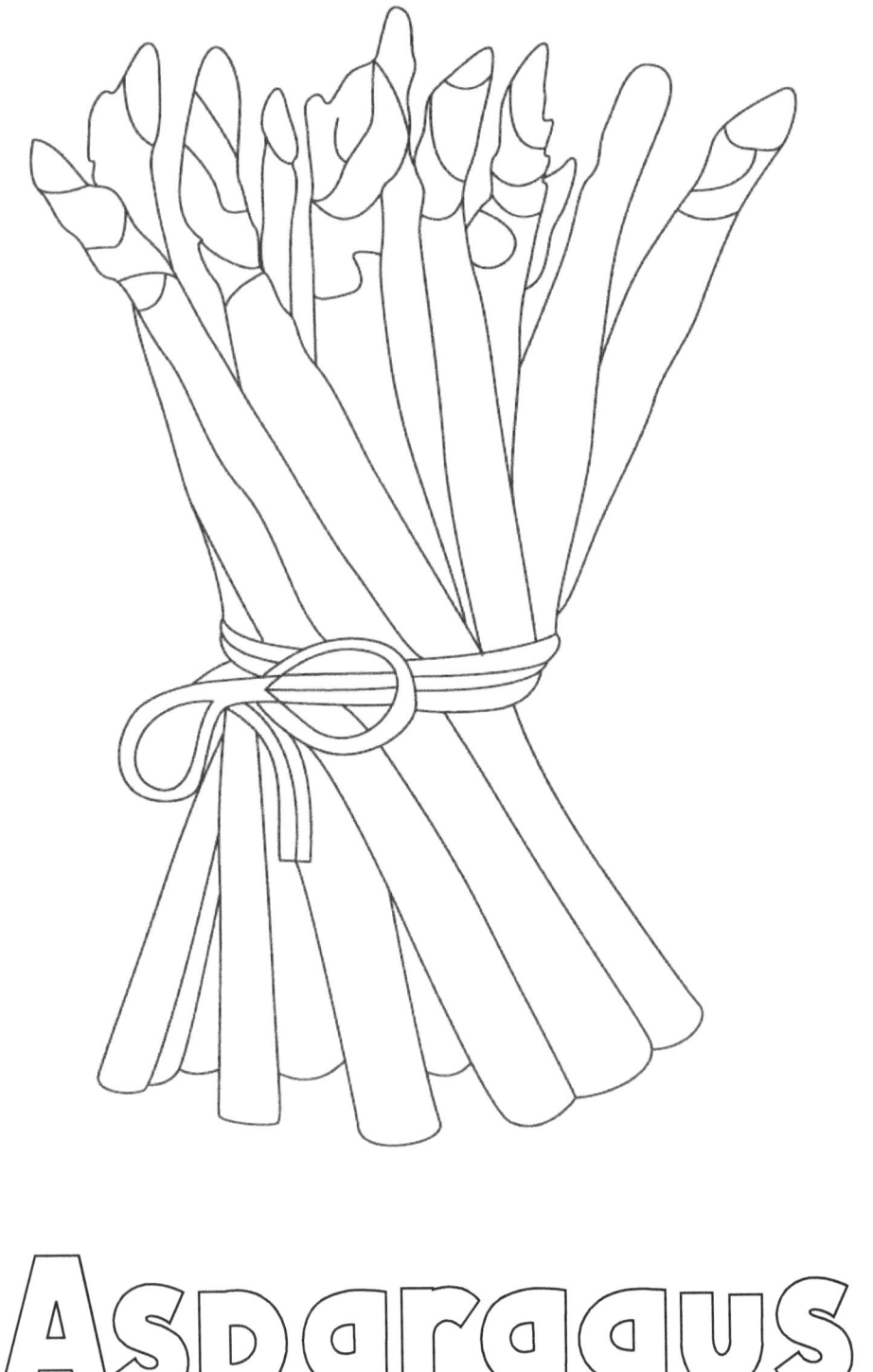

Asparagus

Asparagus is good for health because it is low in calories and rich in vitamins, minerals, and antioxidants, supporting digestive health, promoting heart health, and aiding in weight loss.

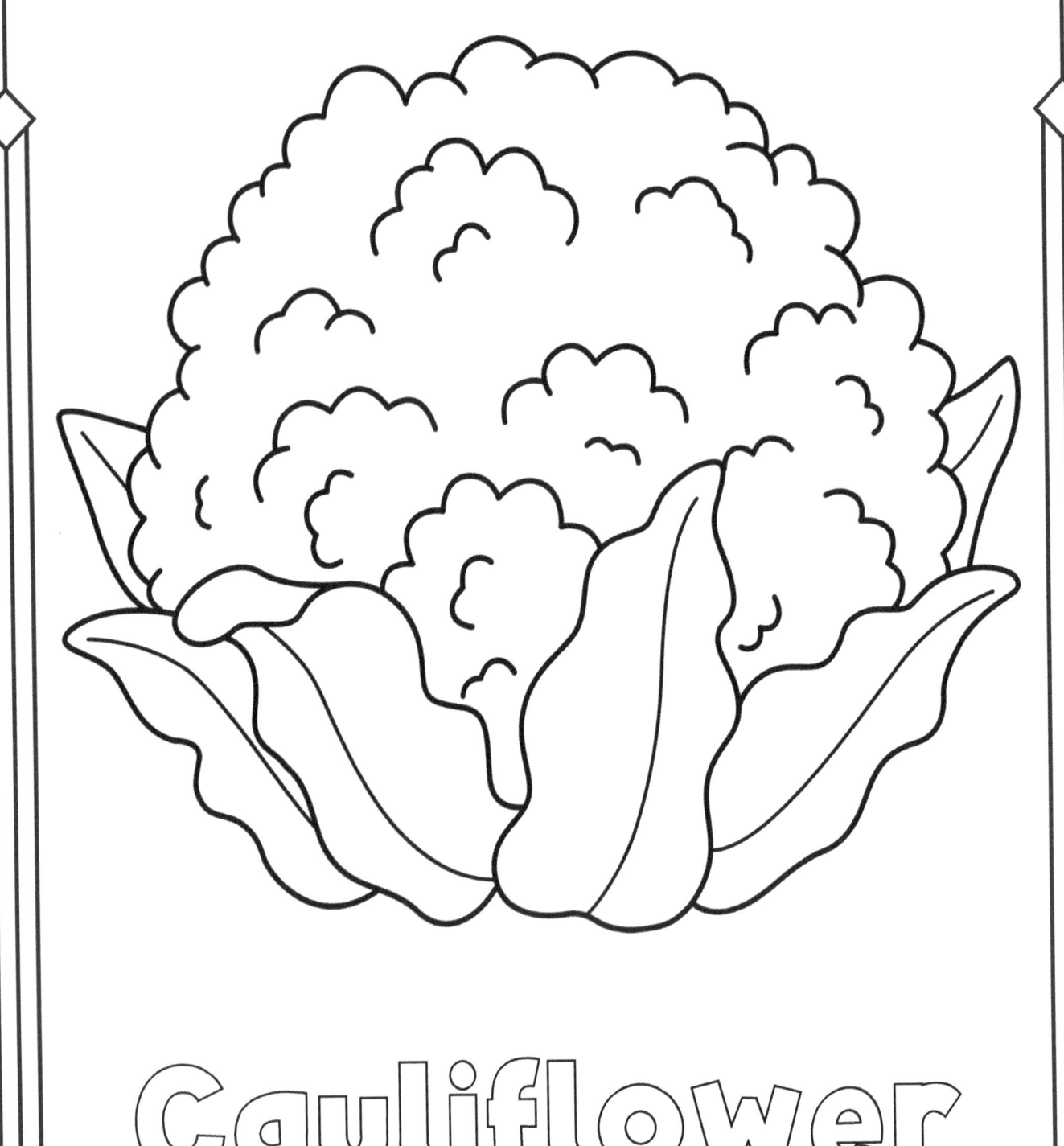

Cauliflower

When it comes to nutrition, cauliflower is a superstar. It's high in vitamins C and K, and is also a good source of folate, which supports cell growth and is essential during pregnancy. Cauliflower is fat-free and cholesterol-free. And it's low in sodium.

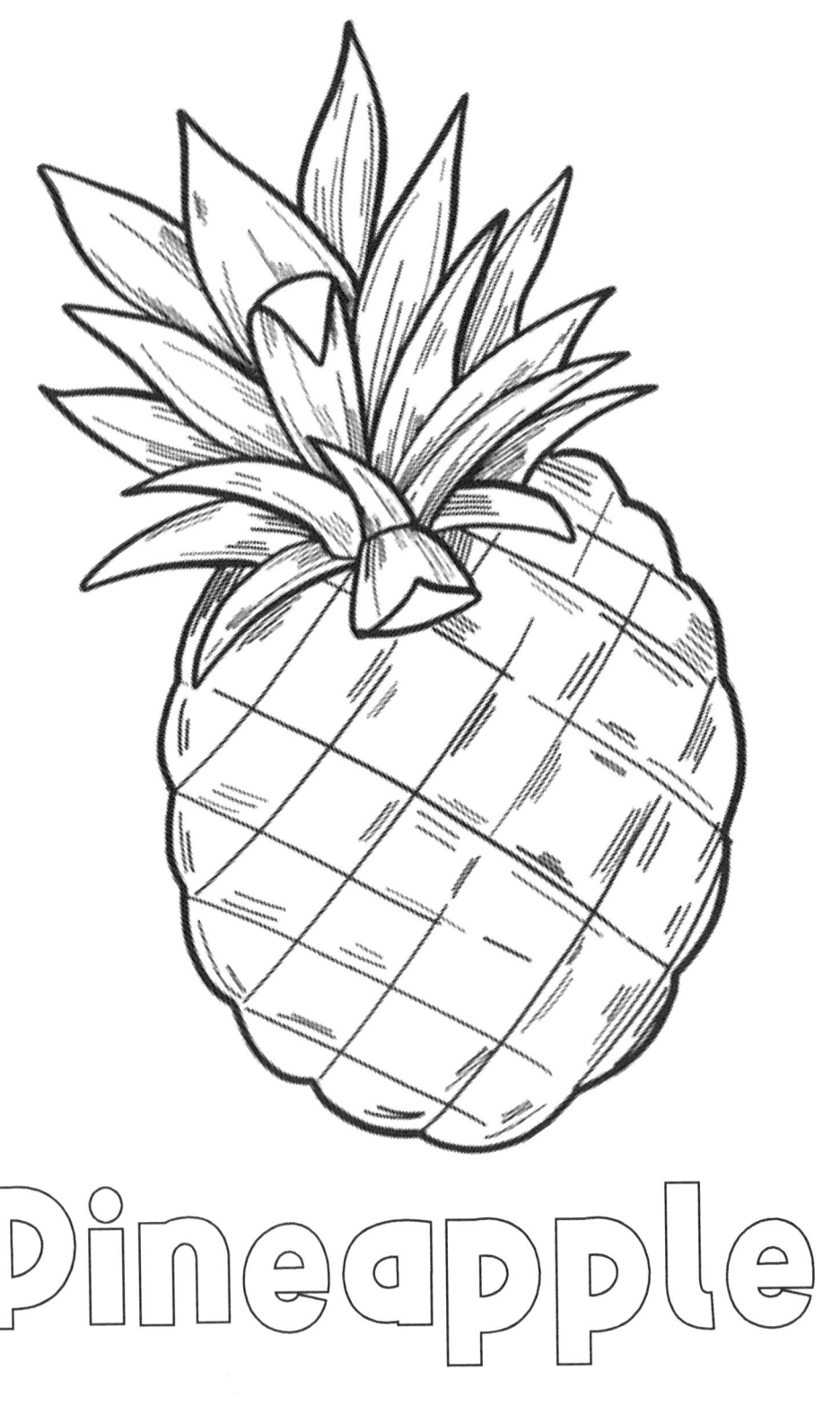

Pineapple

Pineapple is good for health because it is rich in vitamin C, enzymes, and antioxidants, supporting digestion, immune function, and bone health.

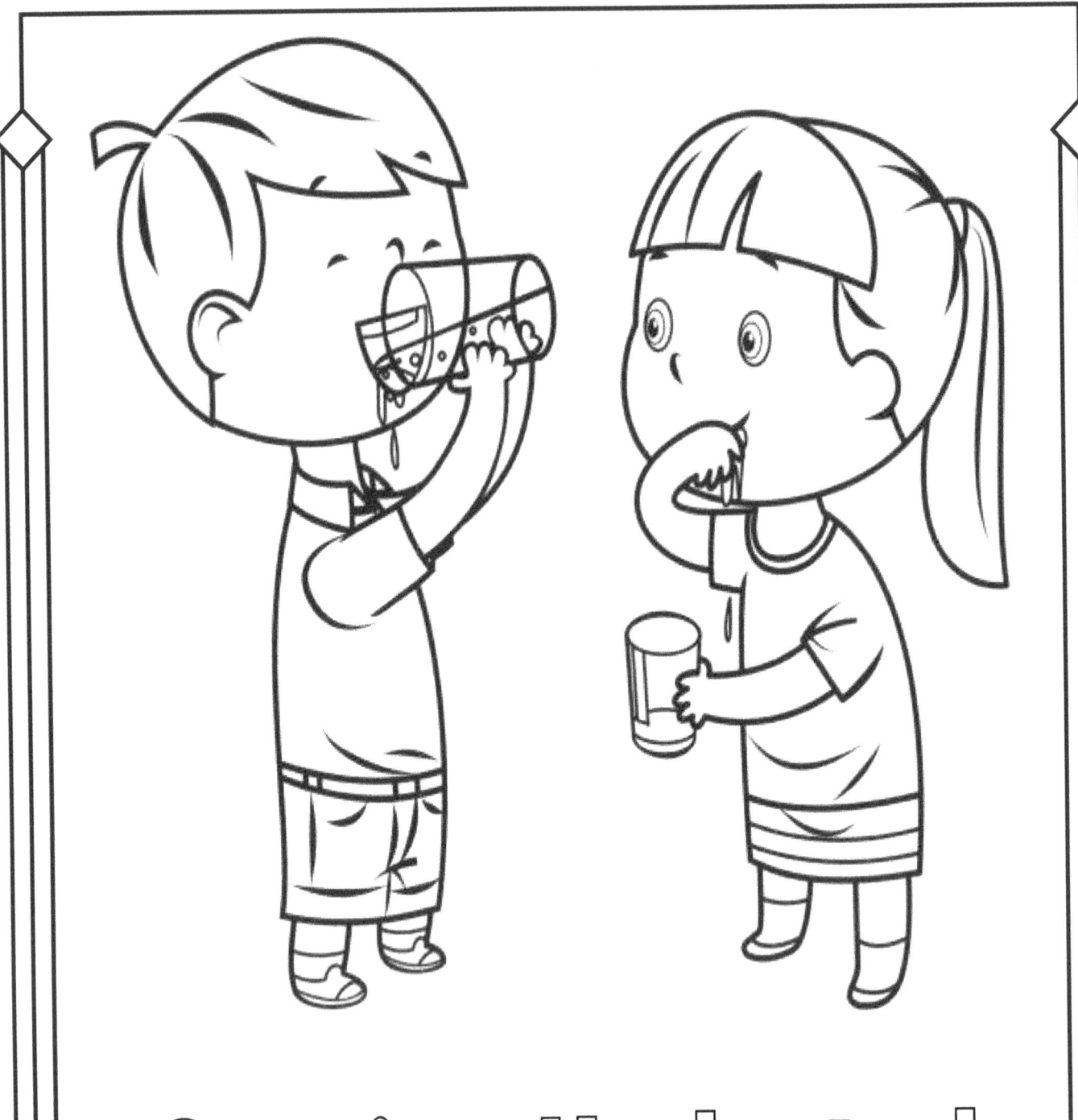

Staying Hydrated

Water is vital to our health. It plays a key role in many of our body's functions, including bringing nutrients to cells, getting rid of wastes, protecting joints and organs, and maintaining body temperature. Water should almost always be your go-to beverage.

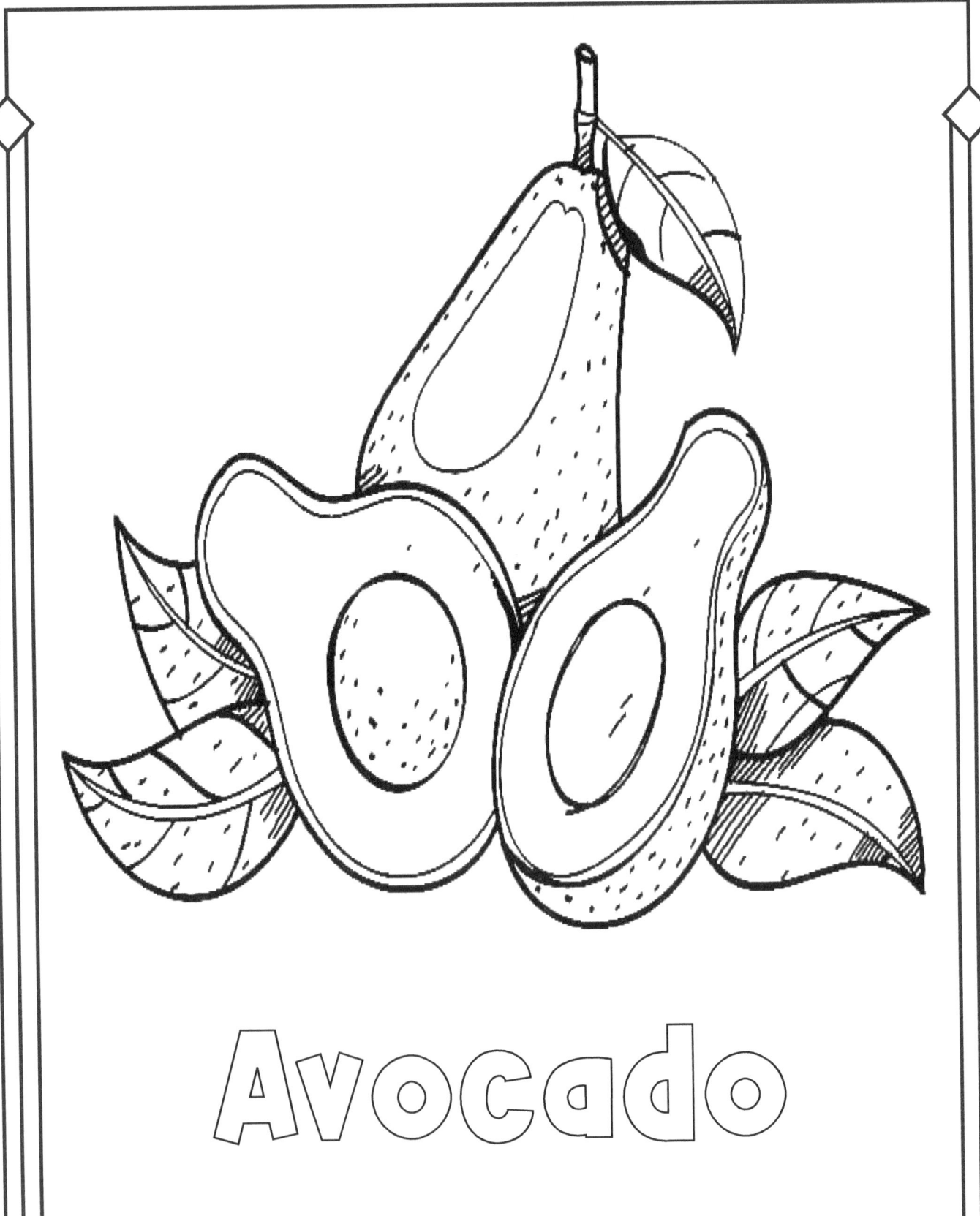

Avocado

Avocado is good for health because it is rich in healthy fats, vitamins, and antioxidants, supporting heart health, promoting skin health, and aiding weight management.

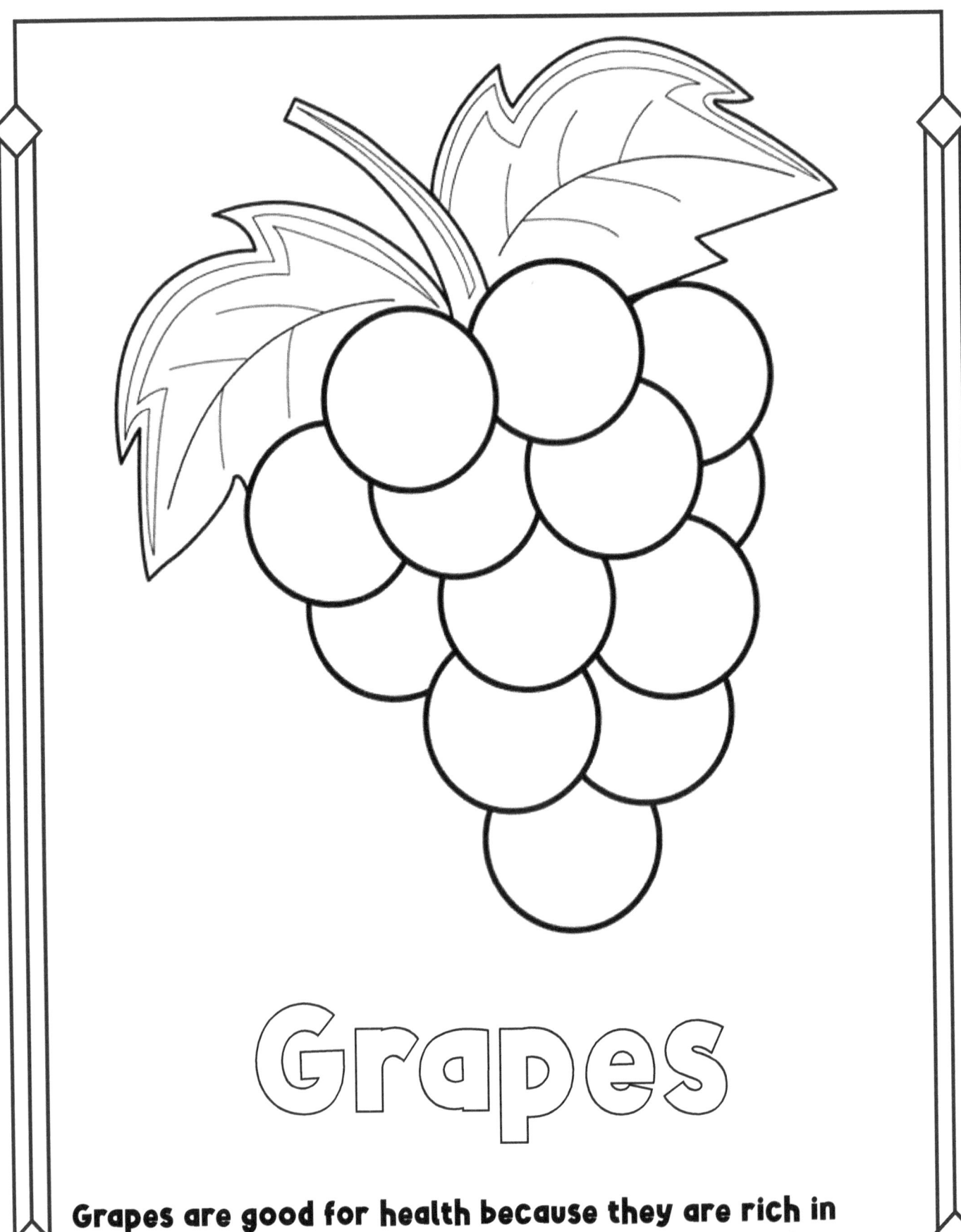

Grapes

Grapes are good for health because they are rich in antioxidants, vitamins, and minerals, supporting heart health, boosting immunity, and promoting healthy aging.

www.ingramcontent.com/pod-product-compliance
Lightning Source LLC
Chambersburg PA
CBHW080550030426
42337CB00024B/4827